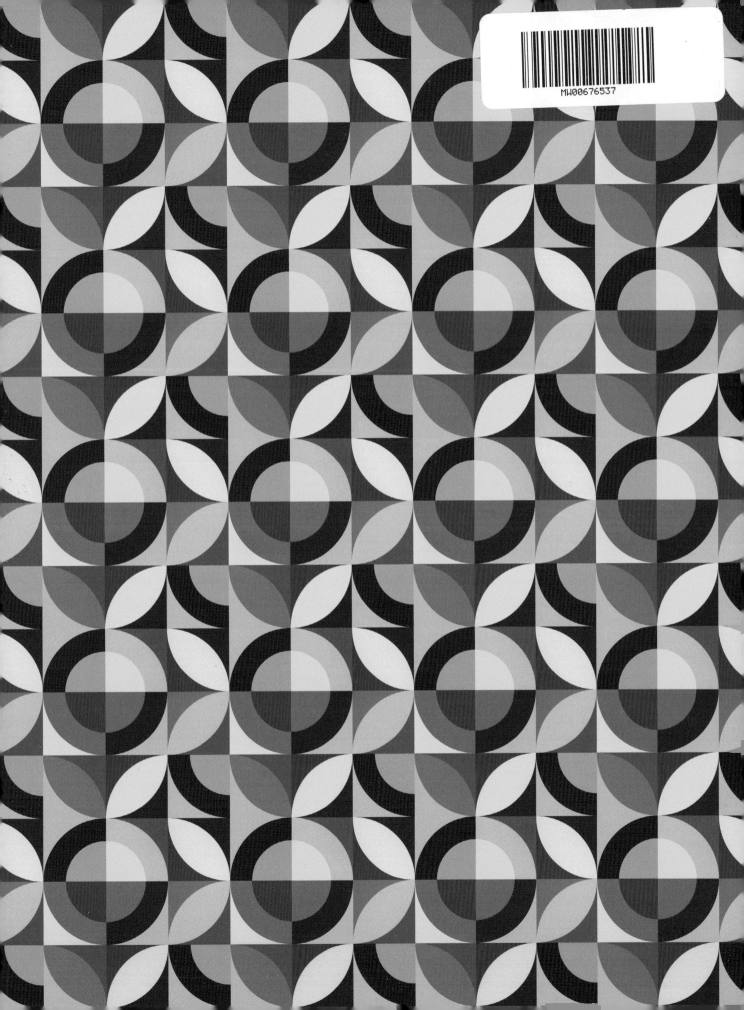

THAT BOWL LIFE

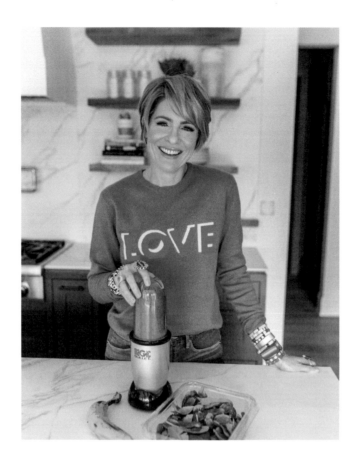

NOT A CHEF? NEITHER AM I.

Beth Chappo is a wife, mother, lifestyle blogger, and accidental cook residing in Zionsville, Indiana. Her love of cooking got a jumpstart after having her son, Calvin, as she was motivated to eat healthy not only for herself but for her family, too. She spent those first few postpartum weeks with a baby wrapped around her and a shortage of hands. The B O W L proved to be super helpful when eating (a.k.a. shoveling her food with the 5 minutes she had available) one-handed. She shares her cooking journey on Instagram with her community of non-cook, one-handed, no time to spare, desire to eat healthy, #bowlievers.

THAT BOWL LIFE

BETH CHAPPO

Photography by Shelly Johnson and Ashley Wittmer

Book Creation by Brunch'd
Photography by Shelly Johnson and Ashley Wittmer
Cover and Interior Design by Megan Wilcop
Edited by Angela McColgin
Food styling by Chung Chow

ISBN 978-1-7344864-0-7

First Edition

Library of Congress Control Number: 2020901899

For That Bowl Life merchandise and more, visit Beth at
www.seersuckerandsaddlesblog.com

TO JOHNNY, CHASE, CAMPBELL, AND CALVIN

Thank you for your endless love, support, and inspiration.
Thank you for humoring me by eating endless bowls of quinoa and cauliflower rice.
You four are what fuel my soul. This one's for you!

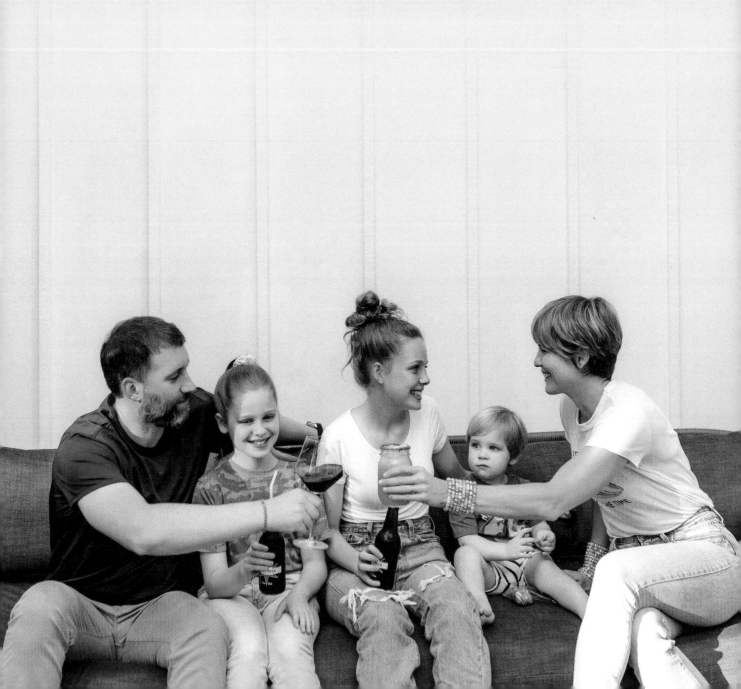

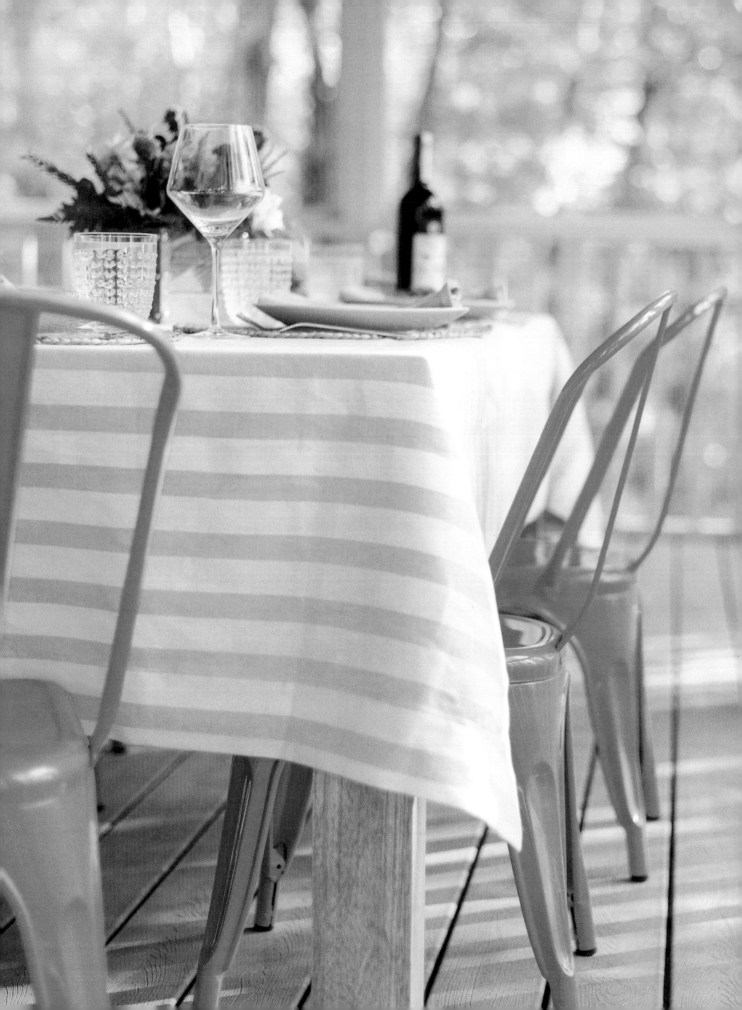

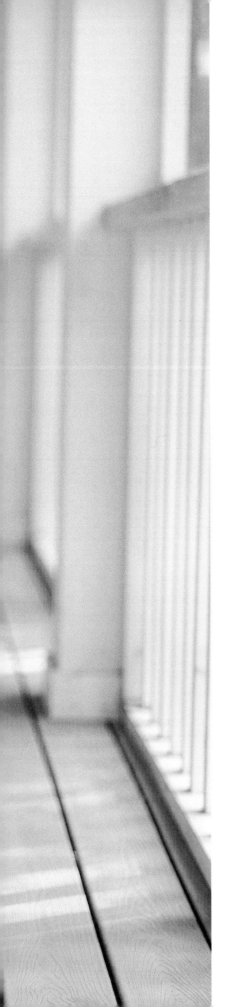

CONTENTS

INTRODUCTION

When I think of myself and cooking, I still do N O T claim to be a chef by any stretch of the imagination. But I have found the parallels between being a fashion blogger and, let's say, a V E R Y casual cook. I get creative, I go with what I like, and I always play by my own rules. I combine things others may find odd, and I'm not afraid to food mix like I print mix—I see you leopard and stripes. I find fun nourishing myself and my fam with the good stuff. And if you ask me, there's no better way to combine, mix, and enjoy your food than in a big ol' bowl!

I invite you to join me in the kitchen and do so with zero hesitation or intimidation. Know that what you'll find in these pages are eats that are easy, healthy, precision-lacking, and flavor-filled. These meals were prepped and shot in my fave space in our home, the kitchen. My hope is that you get in the kitchen and make these dishes for yourself, your friends, and your family, with boatloads of love and laughter.

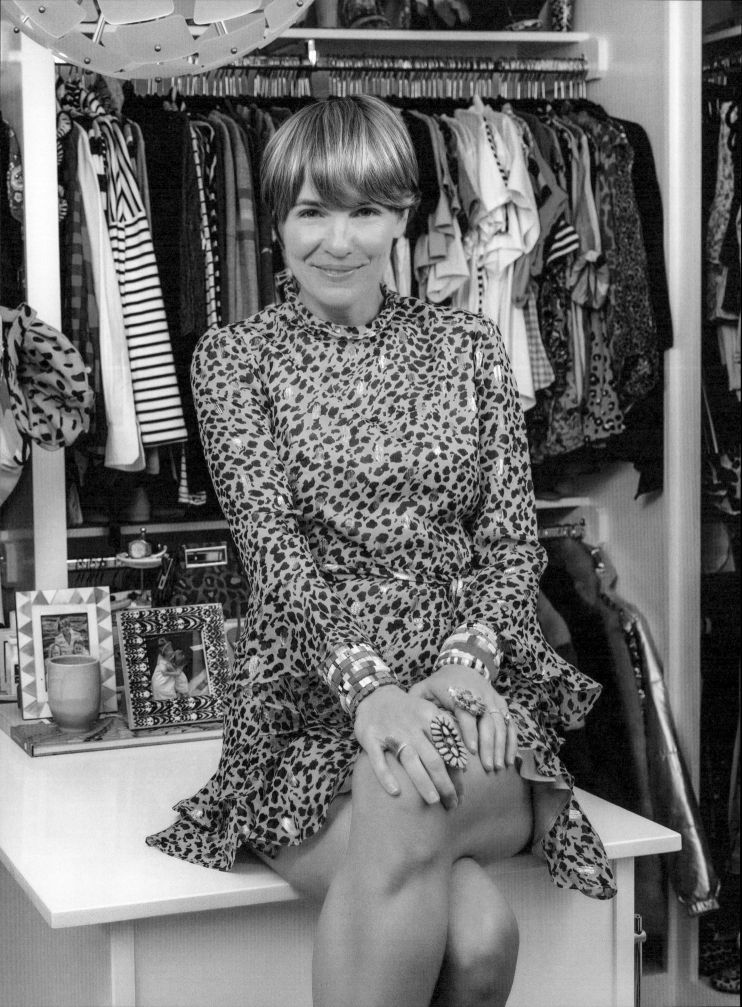

IT'S THE HAULS Y'ALL

TRADER JOE'S HAUL

These are my go-to's when I hit up Trader Joe's. On every trip, I find a new gem or two, but these items are my Trader Joe's staples.

Fruits

- Apples
- Bananas
- Fresh Berries (raspberries, strawberries, blueberries)
- Dried Fruit—I L O V E the Chili Lime Mango!
- Mixed Berry Blend (frozen)
- Tropical Fruit Blend (frozen)

Proteins

- Chicken Breasts, Chicken Tenderloins, Ground Turkey
- Deli Oven Roasted Turkey
- Fresh Hard-Cooked Peeled Eggs
- Sirloin Steak Tips
- Sweet Apple Chicken Sausage
- Uncooked Wild Argentinian Red Shrimp (frozen)

Dairy

- Greek Yogurt
- Cottage Cheese
- Crumbled Feta Cheese
- Goat Cheese
- Shaved Parmesan Cheese
- Crumbled Blue Cheese

Veggies

- Arugula
- Baby Spinach
- Bell Peppers
- Broccoli Florets
- Brussels Sprouts (whole or shaved)
- Riced Cauliflower
- Sweet Potatoes
- Cauliflower Gnocchi (frozen)
- Mashed Cauliflower (frozen)

Grains

- Ezekiel Bread
- Gluten Free Bread
- Microwaveable Brown Rice (frozen)
- Microwaveable Quinoa (frozen)
- Vegetable Fried Rice (frozen)
- Tortillas (corn or flour)

Snacks

- Horseradish Hummus
- Boom Chicka Pop
- Roasted Plantain Chips

Pantry Staples

- Black Beans—all the beans, for that matter.
- Canned Corn
- Petite Diced Tomatoes
- Marinated Artichokes
- Hot & Spicy Dill Pickle Chips
- Salsa Verde
- Sriracha Ranch Dressing
- Coconut Aminos
- Olive Oil
- Coconut Oil
- Avocado Oil
- Everything but the Bagel Sesame Seasoning Blend
- Chili Lime Seasoning Blend

In-a-Pinch Meals

- Chicken Enchiladas Verde
- Chicken Fried Rice
- Mandarin Chicken—grab two while you're at it!

COSTCO HAUL

Full disclosure, this is Johnny's errand. But with this list, he's able to snag all my faves!

Fresh Produce

- Bananas
- Bell Peppers
- Blueberries
- Dates
- Pineapple
- Strawberries
- Broccoli Florets
- Brussels Sprouts
- Butternut Squash Spirals
- Cauliflower Rice
- Romaine Hearts
- Salad Mixes
- Spinach

Proteins

- Eggs
- Greek Yogurt
- Filet Mignon
- Grass Fed Ground Beef
- Kirkland White Albacore Tuna
- Organic Chicken
- Organic Ground Turkey
- Salami
- Salmon

Pantry Staples

- Everything Bagel Seasoning
- Weber Grill Seasoning
- Crunchmaster Multi-Grain Crackers
- Granola

- Grass Fed Beef Jerky
- Skinny Pop
- Basil Pesto
- Canned Black Beans
- Kodiak Cakes Protein Pancake Mix
- Orgain Organic Protein Powder
- Organic Tomato Sauce
- Organic Jack's Cantina Salsa
- Seeds of Change Quinoa and Brown Rice—look for the orange package.
- Avocado Oil Spray
- Kirkland Coconut Oil
- Kirkland Olive Oil
- Parchment Paper

AMAZON HAUL

For my big-ticket items — a.k.a. kitchen gear and bulk staples — always Amazon.

- Magic Bullet Blender
- Vitamix Blender
- Hurom Slow Juicer
- BCAA Powder
- Vital Proteins

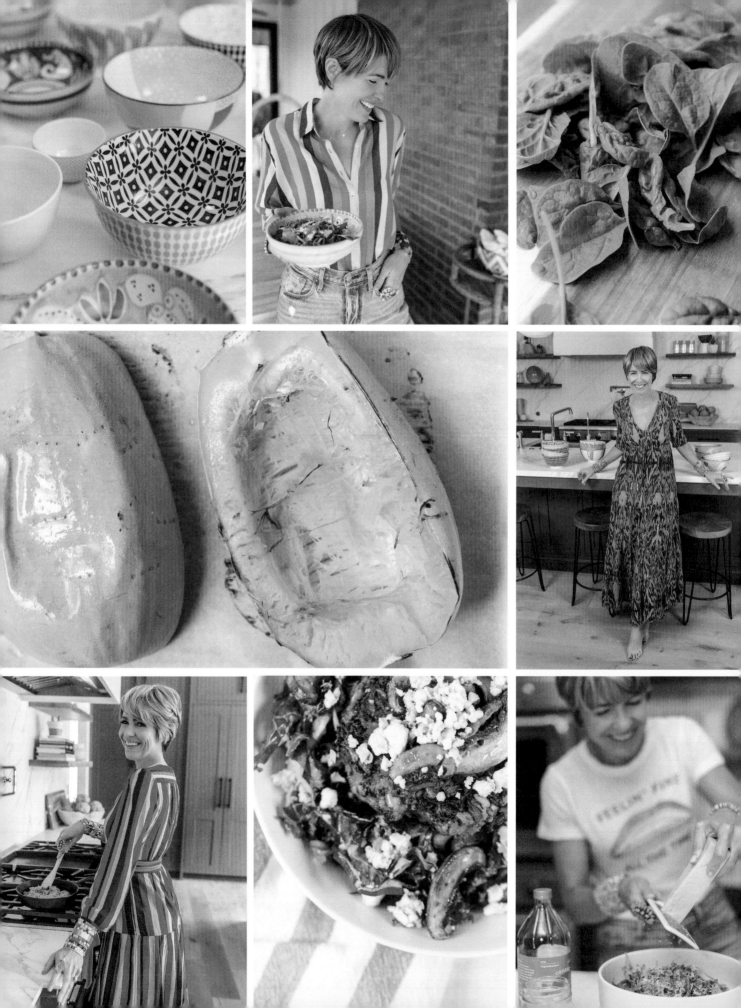

LET'S BUILD A BOWL, SHALL WE?

I approach my closet and getting dressed for the day, the same way I approach meals in my kitchen. When I put together an outfit, I always start with that one perfect piece. It might be uber flattering jeans, flashy and fun sneaks, or the bodysuit that pairs perfectly with everything. In the kitchen, I know that the perfect ingredient, a.k.a. cauliflower rice, flatters E V E R Y dish and pairs PERFECTLY with everything: chicken, beef, tofu, veggies. Then, I spruce up my bowl with, say, for instance, some Sriracha ranch, or a hefty wrist stack, if you follow my drift. In my closet, I look for pieces I'm loving, and in my kitchen, I look for flavors I'm craving, and I build upon it. I always stay open-minded, flexible, and ready to make it work. And that's the beauty of the bowl! You simply can't go wrong.

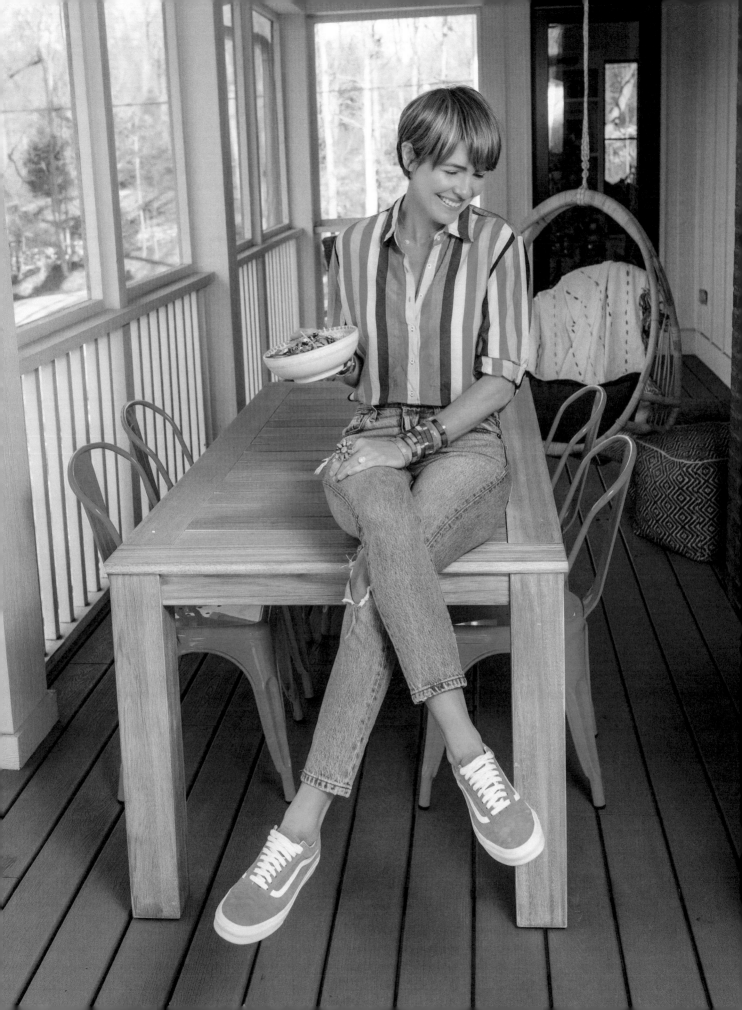

Chapter One

THAT
LOW-CARB
LIFE

Trying to keep those carbs in check?
These are the eats for you!

SEERSUCKER CHICKEN

Get familiar with it! This chicken is a great protein base and can make a cameo
in pretty much any bowl.

Ingredients

Boneless, skinless chicken
breasts or chicken tenderloins

Olive oil

Everything bagel seasoning

Grill seasoning

Parmesan cheese, finely grated

Directions

1. Preheat oven to 425° F and line a baking sheet with parchment paper.

2. In a small bowl, mix generous palmfuls of bagel seasoning, grill seasoning, and parm.

3. Drizzle chicken with olive oil, so seasoning mixture sticks.

4. Toss chicken with seasoning mixture until it is heavily coated on both sides. Don't skimp on this step. The seasoning mix will give the chicken a low-carb crust.

5. Place chicken on baking sheet and bake chicken tenderloins for 15-20 minutes or chicken breasts for 25-30 minutes, until cooked through. Flip chicken halfway through, so it gets crunchy on both sides.

Beth's Tip

This chicken is a great protein base for any bowl or
serve it with a side of *All Day Everyday Arugula* (pg 19).
Cook extra chicken and reheat in the oven or a frying pan.
#leftoversarelife

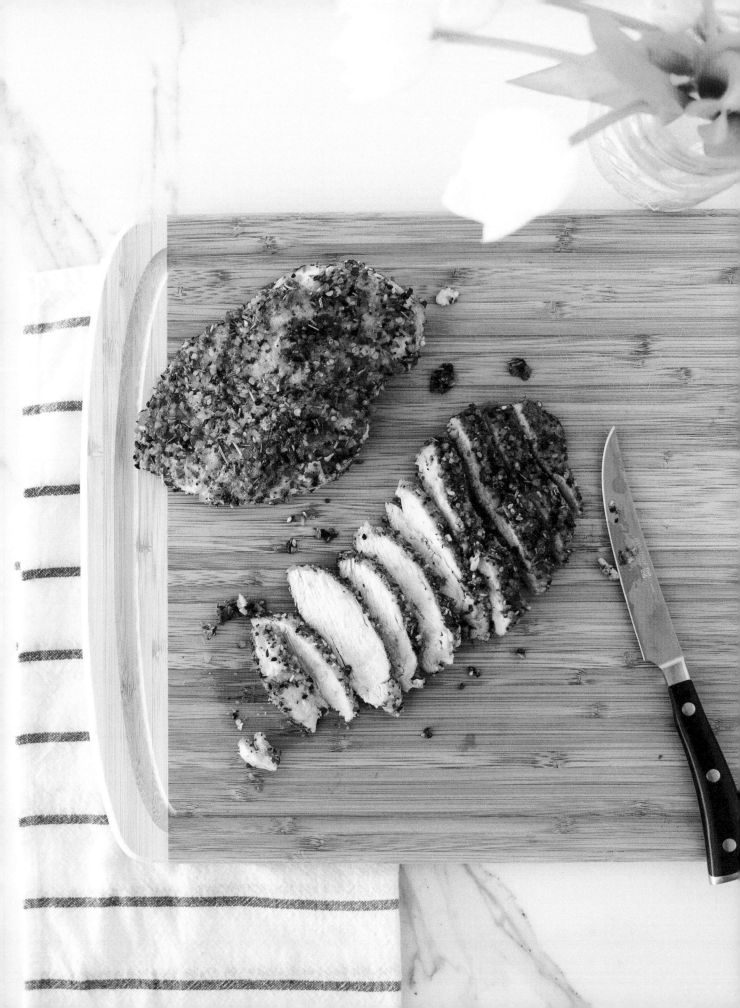

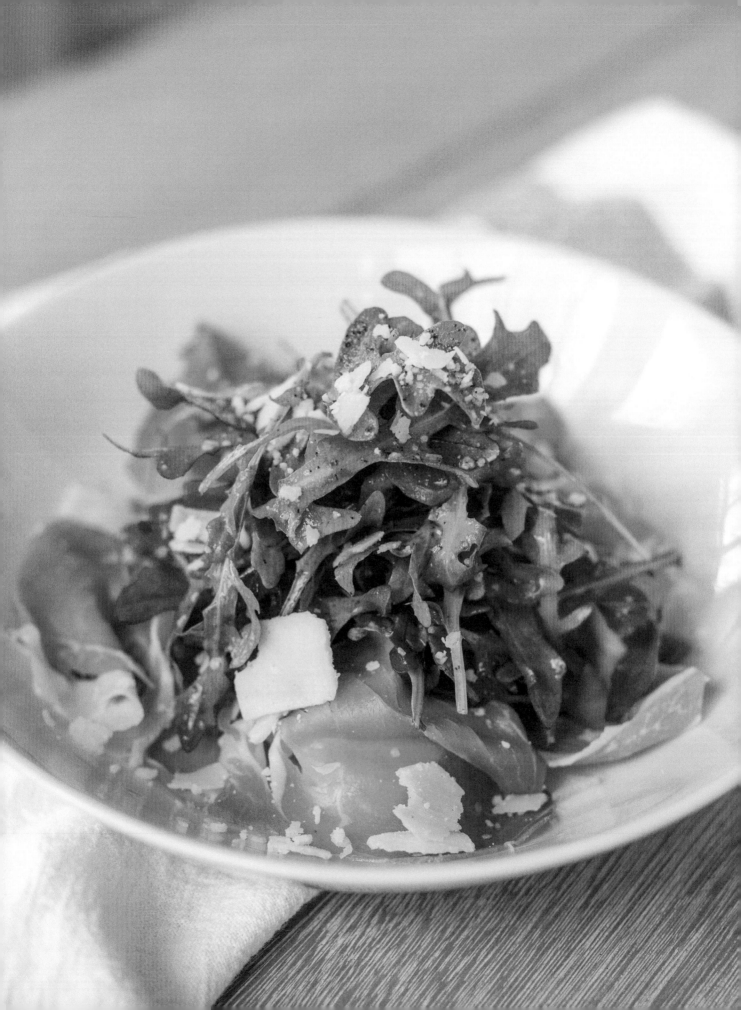

ALL DAY EVERYDAY ARUGULA

Trust me when I say this baby accompanies all bowls! And, it takes two secs to make.

Ingredients

Arugula

Olive oil or avocado oil

Lemon juice or apple cider vinegar—I love both equally!

Everything bagel seasoning or celery salt and black pepper

Parmesan cheese, finely grated

Optional: Prosciutto—add if you need a protein boost.

Directions

1. Toss the arugula with oil, 2-3 capfuls of lemon juice or vinegar. Season with bagel seasoning or celery salt and pepper and parm.

2. If using prosciutto, layer a plate with prosciutto slices.

3. Build your bowl: put a big ol' mound of arugula on top of the prosciutto or put the arugula mix on top of your favorite bowl and E N J O Y!

BLACK AND BLUE BOWL

Hearty and chock full of flavor, this bowl packs a protein punch.

Ingredients

Avocado oil

Sirloin steak tips

Chili lime seasoning

Mushrooms

Arugula

Lemon juice

Everything bagel seasoning

Blue cheese crumbles

Directions

1. Heat avocado oil in a skillet over medium-high heat.

2. Season steak tips heavily with chili lime.

3. Once the skillet is nice and hot, add meat in a single layer. Listen for the sizzle. Cook steak for 2-3 minutes per side, depending on temperature preference. Transfer meat to a plate.

4. In the same skillet, add sliced mushrooms and sauté for 3-4 minutes. Season with chili lime.

5. In a separate bowl, toss the arugula with avocado oil, lemon juice, and bagel seasoning.

6. Build your bowl: layer steak on top of arugula, top with sautéed mushrooms, and blue cheese crumbles and E N J O Y.

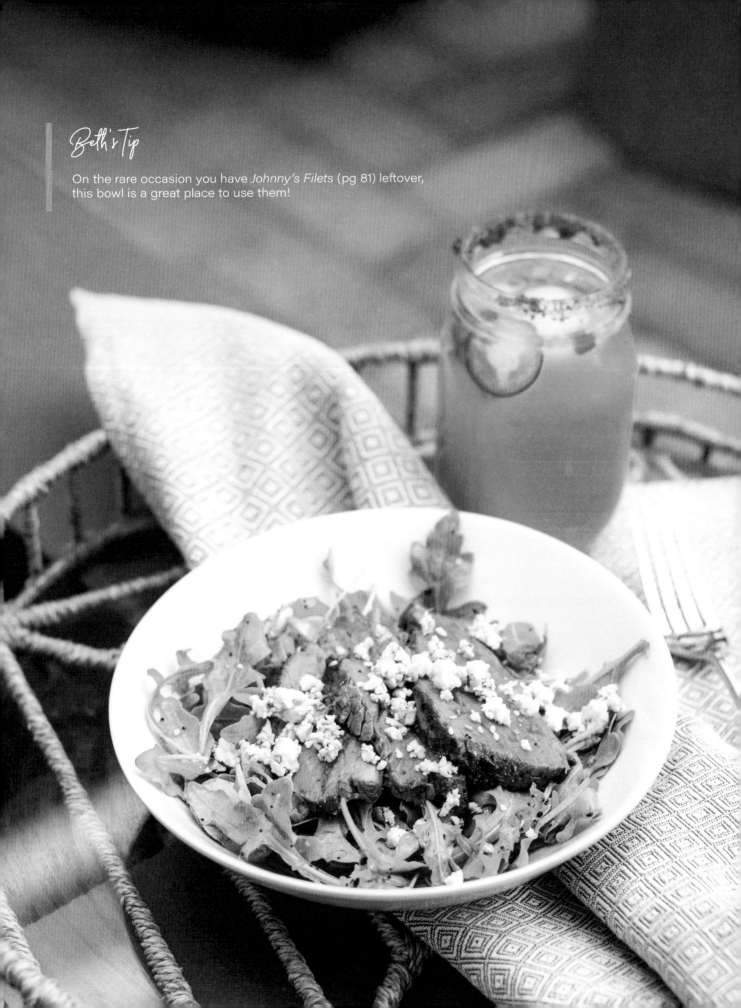

Beth's Tip

On the rare occasion you have *Johnny's Filets* (pg 81) leftover, this bowl is a great place to use them!

EGGPLANT PARM STACKS

Whipped this baby up and fell in love with it all in the same night.

Ingredients

Sneaky Veggie Tomato Sauce

Marinara sauce

Baby spinach

Olive oil

1-2 cloves of garlic, minced

Salt and pepper

Italian seasoning

Eggplant Stacks

2 medium eggplants

Everything bagel seasoning

Grill seasoning

Olive oil

Parmesan cheese, finely grated

Mozzarella cheese, shredded

Zucchini noodles

Directions

Make the Sneaky Veggie Tomato Sauce

1. Add marinara sauce and a big ol' handful of baby spinach to a blender and blend until smooth.

2. Heat olive oil in a saucepan over medium-high heat. Add minced garlic, and do a quick sauté. Add blended marinara sauce. Season to taste with salt, pepper, and italian seasoning.

3. Bring sauce to a boil and then lower heat to keep the sauce at a simmer. While your sauce simmers away, work on your eggplant and zucchini noodles.

Make the Eggplant Stacks

1. Peel the eggplant and slice into ½-inch-thick circles. Lay eggplant circles on paper towels and sprinkle with salt. Let sit for 5-10 minutes to remove excess moisture.

2. In a small bowl, mix generous palmfuls of bagel seasoning, grill seasoning, and parm to create "breading" mixture.

3. Dry eggplant slices with paper towels, drizzle with olive oil and coat each side with "breading" mixture.

4. Heat olive oil in a skillet over medium-high heat, making sure there is enough oil to coat the bottom of the pan. Fry eggplant slices for about 2 minutes each side until golden brown. Drain eggplant on paper towels.

5. Once all eggplant is fried, add zucchini noodles to the same pan and lightly sauté. Season to taste with salt and pepper and toss with half of the *Sneaky Veggie Tomato Sauce.*

6. On a foil-lined baking sheet, create your eggplant stacks in this order: eggplant, *Sneaky Veggie Tomato Sauce*, and mozzarella. Repeat.

7. Pop eggplant stacks under the broiler just long enough to melt the cheese.

8. Build your bowl: serve eggplant stacks with zucchini noodles and C H O W.

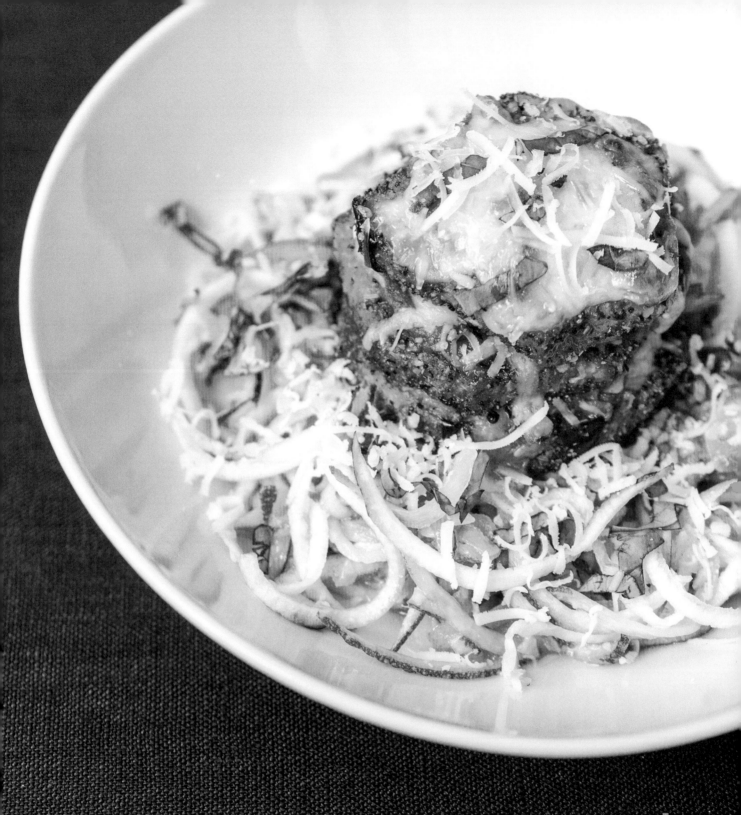

Beth's Tip

Need a protein boost? Add *Seersucker Chicken* (pg 16).
Feeling extra frisky? Add a pile of *All Day Everyday Arugula* (pg 19).

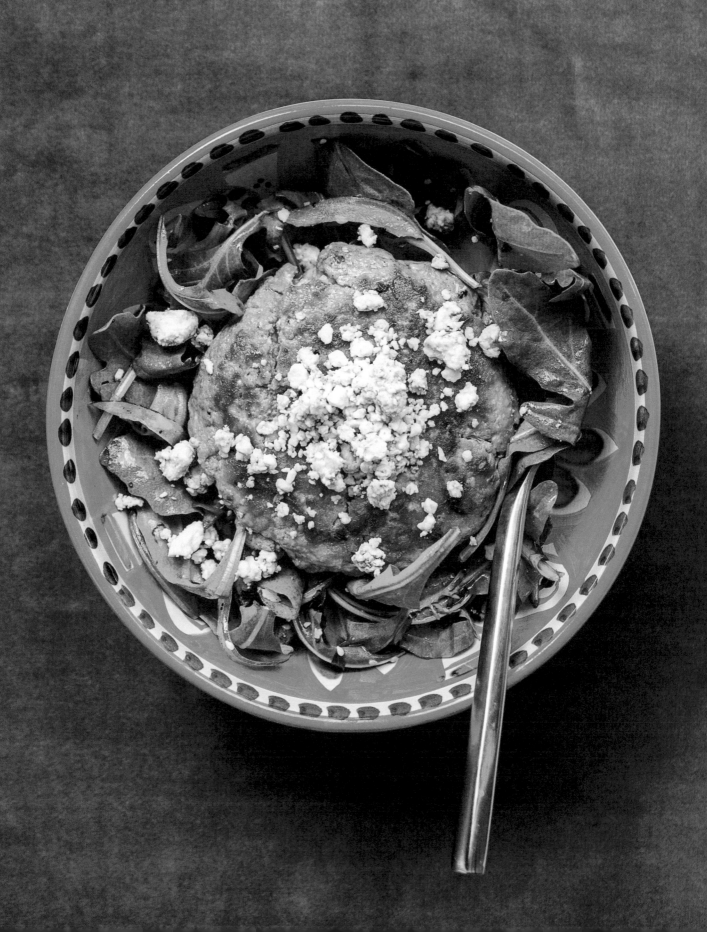

BUFFALO BLUE TURKEY BURGER

Just because it's low-carb, doesn't mean it has to be boring. This bad boy ain't boring!

Ingredients

1 pound ground turkey

2-3 tablespoons louisiana-style hot sauce

½ cup blue cheese crumbles

Avocado oil

All Day Everyday Arugula
(pg 19)

Directions

1. In a large bowl, get your hands dirty and combine ground turkey, hot sauce, and blue cheese crumbles.

2. Form burger mix into 4 patties. Use your thumb and make a slight indentation in the middle of each patty, which will help the burger hold its shape while cooking.

3. Heat avocado oil in a large skillet over medium-high heat.

4. Cook burgers 4-6 minutes per side, until crispy golden brown on the outside and no longer pink in the middle.

5. Drain burgers on paper towels.

6. Build your bowl: serve burger on top of *All Day Everyday Arugula*, top with blue cheese crumbles, and extra hot sauce. It might be wise to have a tall glass of H2O on hand for this one.

Beth's Tip

Use avocado oil rather than olive oil when cooking at high heat.

THAT EGG ROLL BOWL

She may not look like much, but man, is she!

Ingredients

Sesame oil

1 pound ground turkey or ground pork

1 bag coleslaw mix

1 tablespoon rice wine vinegar

1/4 cup soy sauce

1 tablespoon Sriracha

Sriracha ranch dressing

Sesame seeds

Directions

1. Heat sesame oil in a large skillet over medium-high heat. Brown ground turkey or ground pork until no longer pink, 8-10 minutes.

2. In a separate skillet, heat sesame oil over medium-high heat. Add coleslaw mix and sauté until tender, about 5 minutes.

3. In a small bowl, make a sauce with rice wine vinegar, soy sauce, and Sriracha.

4. Add the sauce and cooked turkey or pork to the coleslaw mix. Stir until combined.

5. Build your bowl: put a big ol' heap of the coleslaw mixture into your bowl. Top with Sriracha ranch and sesame seeds. You can enjoy this bowl now, but it's just as good later. #leftoversarelife

Beth's Tip

Top this bowl with a fried egg, and it's perfect for brunch!

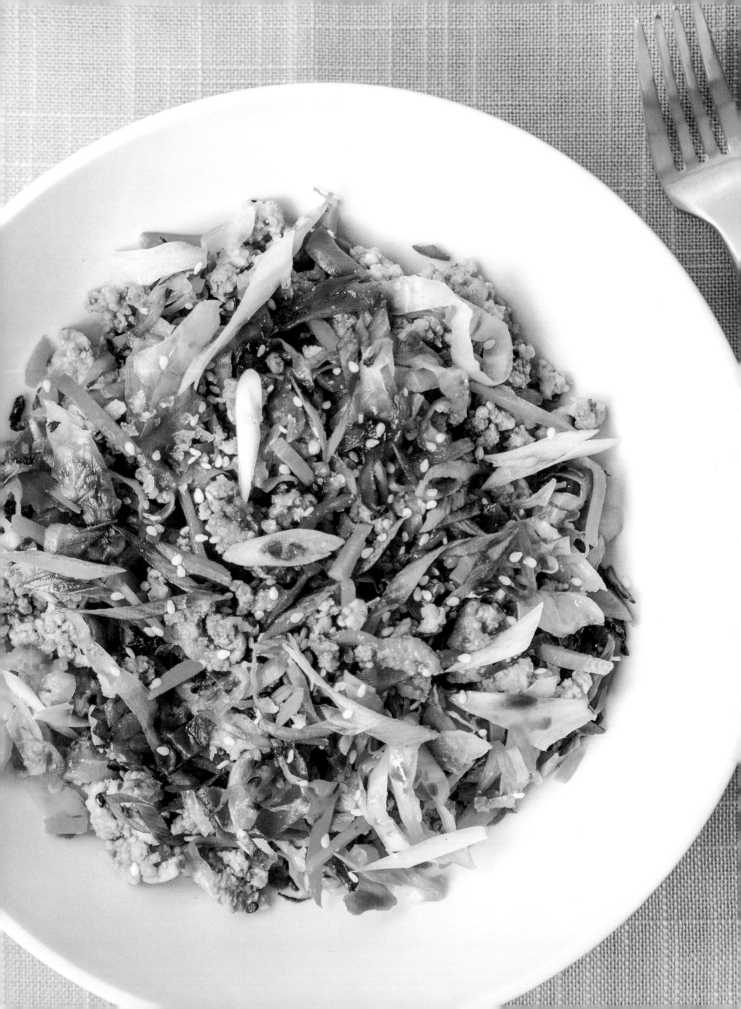

SHRIMP AND CAULIFLOWER GRITS

Blame it on my time in Kentucky. This one has my (low-carb) heart.

Ingredients

Raw shrimp, fresh or frozen

Chili lime seasoning

Avocado oil

Mashed cauliflower, frozen

Goat cheese

Sriracha ranch dressing

Directions

1. If using frozen shrimp, stick it in a colander and thaw by running under cold water for 5-10 minutes. Pat shrimp dry with paper towels.

2. Season shrimp with a boatload of chili lime.

3. Heat avocado oil in a large skillet over medium-high heat. Add shrimp and cook, tossing for 3-4 minutes, until the shrimp is cooked through.

4. Heat avocado oil in a saucepan over medium-high heat. Add frozen mashed cauliflower, **without any additional water**. Stir and heat through.

5. Add a generous amount of goat cheese and stir until combined.

6. Build your bowl: spoon cauliflower grits into a bowl, top with shrimp, and a drizzle of Sriracha ranch and GO. TO. CHOW. TOWN.

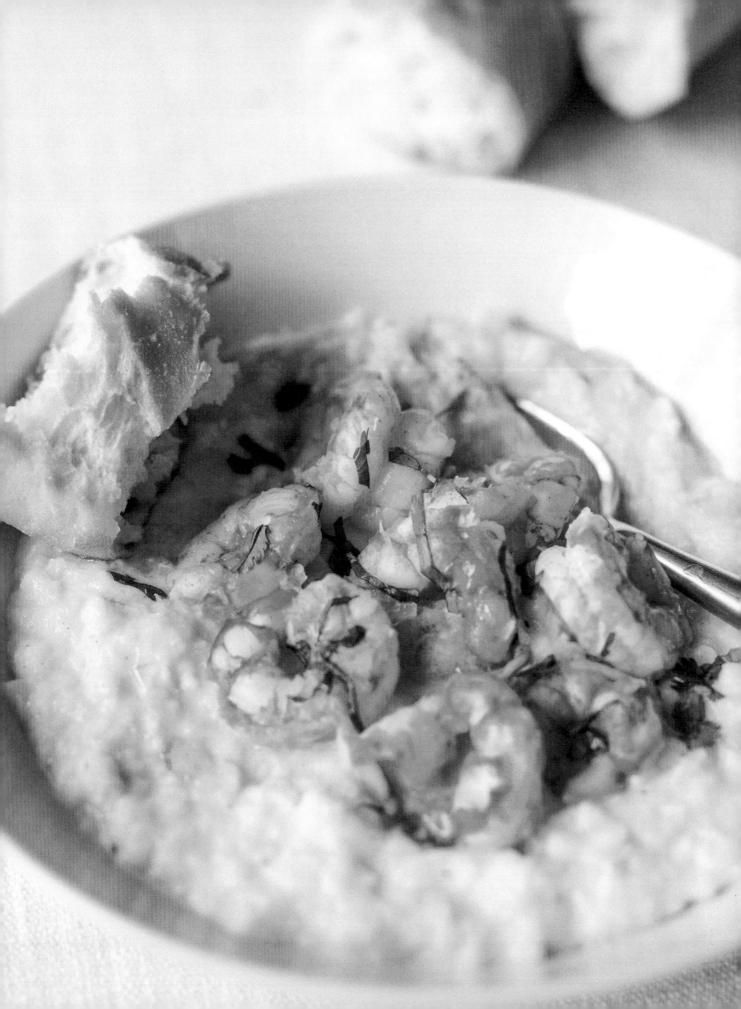

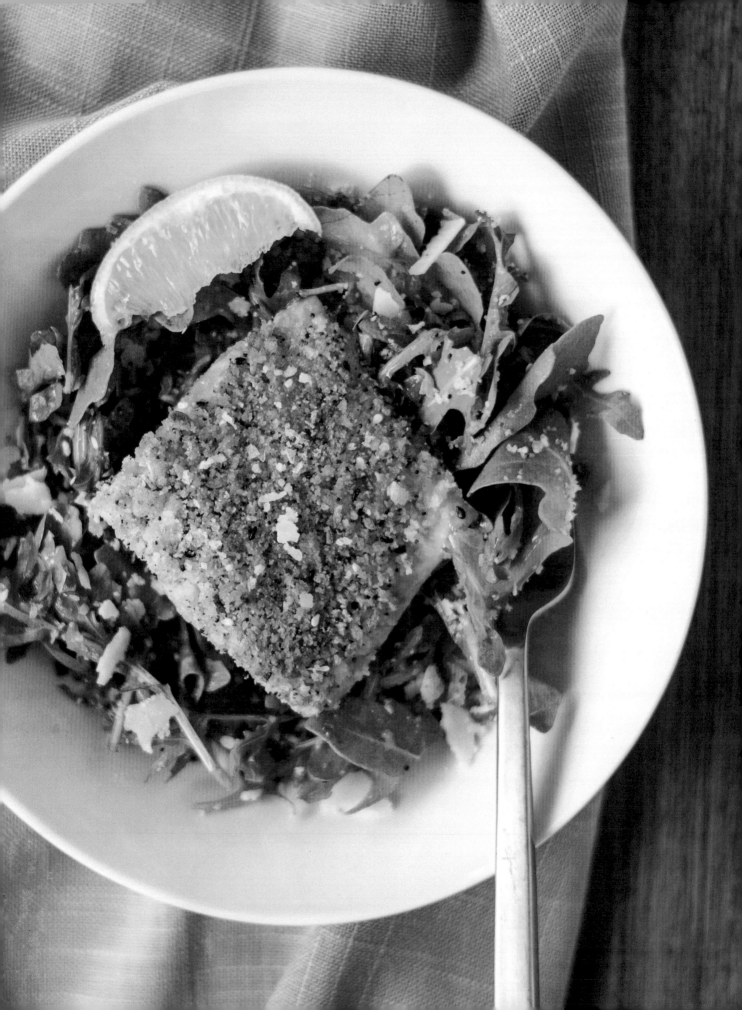

PARMESAN CRUSTED SALMON AND ARUGULA

Fresh and light but chock full of delish delight.

Ingredients

Large salmon fillet

Olive oil

Panko breadcrumbs

Everything bagel seasoning

Parmesan cheese, finely grated

All Day Everyday Arugula
(pg 19)

Directions

1. Preheat oven to 425°F and line a baking sheet with foil.

2. Cut salmon into 6-8 ounce portions (about a hand-width). 2 pounds of salmon will be approximately four fillets.

3. Place salmon on the baking sheet, skin side down, and rub with olive oil.

4. In a small bowl, mix generous palmfuls of panko, bagel seasoning, and parm.

5. Pour the breadcrumb mixture evenly over the salmon to create a crust, patting it down until the top of each fillet is covered.

6. Pop salmon in the oven for about 15 minutes until the crust is golden and the salmon flakes easily with a fork.

7. Build your bowl: serve salmon with *All Day Everyday Arugula*. Voila!

Beth's Tip

Use leftovers for *Ashley's Salmon Salad* (pg 150), and spread the love all week long.

PESTO CHICKEN CAULIFLOWER PIZZA

You won't know it's not the real deal.

Ingredients

Grape or cherry tomatoes

Olive oil

Everything bagel seasoning

Cauliflower pizza crust

Pesto

Parmesan cheese, finely grated

Seersucker Chicken (pg 16)

All Day Everyday Arugula (pg 19)

Directions

1. Preheat oven to 350° F and line a baking sheet with parchment paper.

2. Halve your tomatoes. Toss with a drizzle of olive oil and season with bagel seasoning. Place tomatoes in a single layer on the baking sheet and roast for 15-20 minutes.

3. While the tomatoes are roasting, brush the cauliflower pizza crust with olive oil and place DIRECTLY on the oven rack for about 5 minutes shy of the package directions.

4. Gently remove the crust from the oven. She's fragile. Spread a layer of pesto onto the crust. Top with chicken, roasted tomatoes, and parm.

5. Put pizza back in the oven long enough to melt the cheese.

6. This pairs beautifully with *All Day Everyday Arugula* either on top or on the side. BON APPETIT!

Beth's Tip

Don't have any *Seersucker Chicken* in the fridge?
Grab a rotisserie chicken, and you're good to go! #momhacks

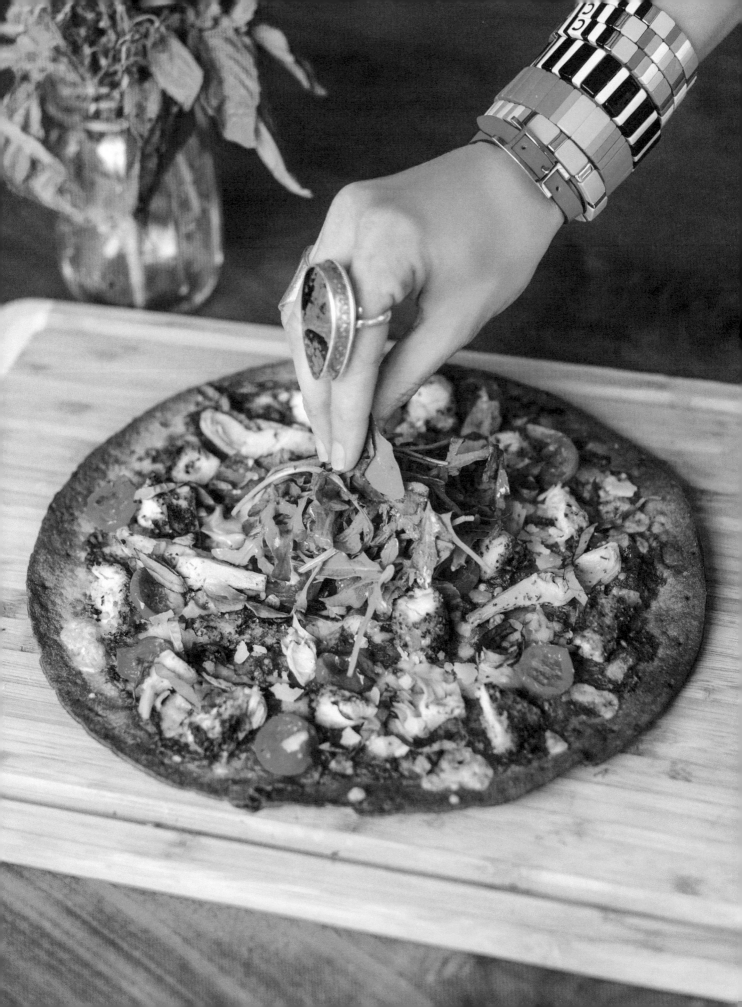

SALSA VERDE CHICKEN

Imagine your favorite dress styled three different ways. Welcome to Salsa Verde Chicken!

Ingredients

Boneless, skinless chicken breasts or chicken tenderloins

1 jar salsa verde

Cauliflower rice

Kale, shredded

Olive oil

Chili lime seasoning

Low-Carb and Tacos:

Sliced avocado

Chili lime seasoning

Feta cheese

Sriracha ranch dressing

Low-carb or regular tortillas

Greek yogurt

Regular Macro:

Brown rice

Black beans

Directions

1. Place chicken in a slowcooker, cover with salsa verde, and stir to coat. Leave a little salsa in the jar for topping your bowl.

2. Cover and cook 4 hours on high or 6 hours on low.

3. When it's almost time to eat, preheat oven to 425°F and line a baking sheet with parchment paper.

4. Add cauliflower rice to one half of the baking sheet and shredded kale to the other half. Drizzle everything with olive oil and season with chili lime.

5. Roast vegetables for 25 minutes.

6. Remove chicken from the slow-cooker and shred into bite-size pieces.

7. Put the shredded chicken back into the crockpot and mix with the sauce.

8. Style your chicken the way that works for you. You can even get adventurous and think outside THE BOWL.

Beth's Tip

Use a hand mixer to perfectly shred your *Salsa Verde Chicken.*

1. LOW-CARB

Fill your bowl with cauliflower rice and top with a heaping pile of *Salsa Verde Chicken*. Top with sliced avocado seasoned with chili lime, roasted kale, feta, salsa verde, and a drizzle of Sriracha ranch.

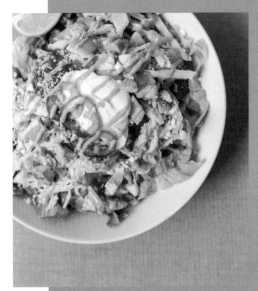

2. THE TACO

Wrap tortillas in a damp paper towel and microwave for 15 seconds. Add all the toppings to your tortilla. I told you this was easy!

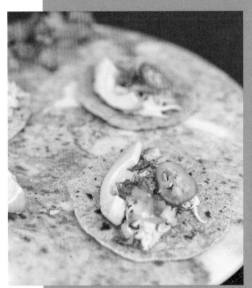

3. REGULAR MACRO

For a regular macro day, swap out the cauliflower rice for brown rice and add some black beans and greek yogurt seasoned with chili lime.

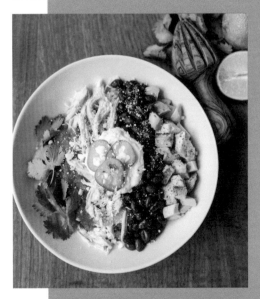

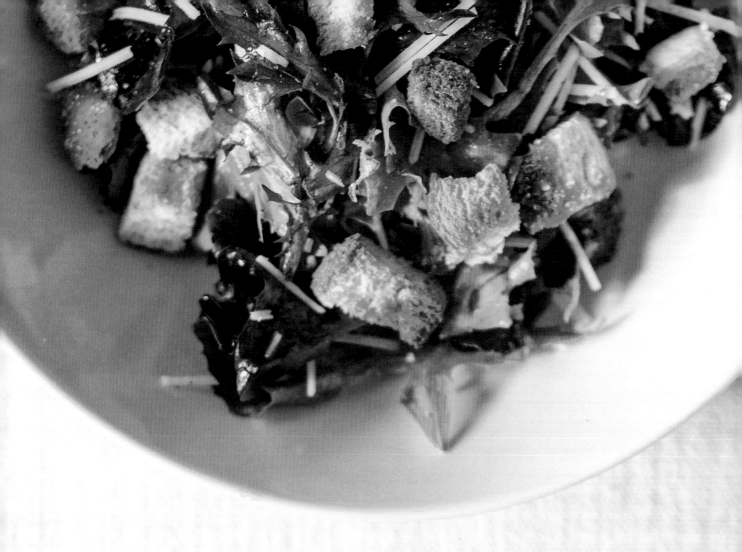

AUNT KITTY

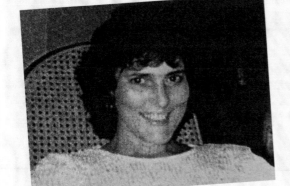

She and my mom have always been exceptionally close. When I was younger, once a month or so, my mom and I would go to her condo in Palm Beach Gardens, Florida, to visit her, my Aunt Eileen, and her little white dog, Lambchop. On every visit, we had this salad in wooden bowls, topped with heaps of Parmesan cheese, and onions, which I would invariably remove. I loved the smell of that salad, the taste, the bowls. I have searched for replicas of those salad bowls and still haven't found any that quite measure up. I didn't realize that "Aunt Kitty Salad" would forever be engrained in my mind, and that it would become one of my favorite bowls, but indeed Aunt Kitty, it is.

AUNT KITTY SALAD

Ingredients

Romaine or spring mix

Apple cider vinegar

Olive oil

Celery salt

Cracked black pepper

Parmesan cheese, shaved

Red onion (optional)

Croutons (optional)

Directions

1. Toss spring mix into a bowl and dress with 2-3 capfuls of apple cider vinegar and a generous drizzle of olive oil.

2. Season with celery salt and cracked black pepper.

3. Build your bowl: top salad with a heap of parm, a little diced red onion, and croutons.

Beth's Tip

Best served in Aunt Kitty's wooden bowls, but any bowl will do.
Hopefully, this dish will bring you as many fond memories as it did me.

SPAGHETTI SQUASH WITH PESTO AND TOMATOES

Pasta lovers, this one's for you!

Ingredients

Spaghetti squash

Olive oil

Grape or cherry tomatoes

Everything bagel seasoning

Pesto

Parmesan cheese, shaved

Seersucker Chicken (pg 16)

Directions

1. Preheat oven to 400°F and line a baking sheet with parchment paper.

2. Using some elbow grease and a heavy-duty knife cut your squash in half from stem to tail. Scoop out the squash guts.

3. Drizzle olive oil over squash and season with salt and pepper.

4. Place the squash halves cut side down on one half of the baking sheet.

5. Add tomatoes to the other half of the baking sheet. Drizzle with olive oil and season with bagel seasoning.

6. Roast for 20 minutes, then remove the baking sheet from the oven and place tomatoes in a bowl.

7. Return squash to the oven and roast for an additional 15-20 minutes. You'll know the squash is done when it is easily pierced with a fork.

8. Use a fork to scrape the squash out of the shell into fine strings. Place shredded squash into a bowl, and mix with pesto.

9. Build your bowl: add pesto dressed spaghetti squash, *Seersucker Chicken*, and roasted tomatoes. Top with shaved parm. EAT 'ER UP!

Beth's Tip

If you're short on time, cook your squash in the microwave. Stab squash all over with a fork. Place whole squash in the microwave and cook in 5-minute intervals, rotating after each interval. Cook for 10-15 minutes until soft. Cut squash in half—watch out it will be H O T—and scoop out the seeds. Use a fork to scrape the squash out of the shell into fine strings.

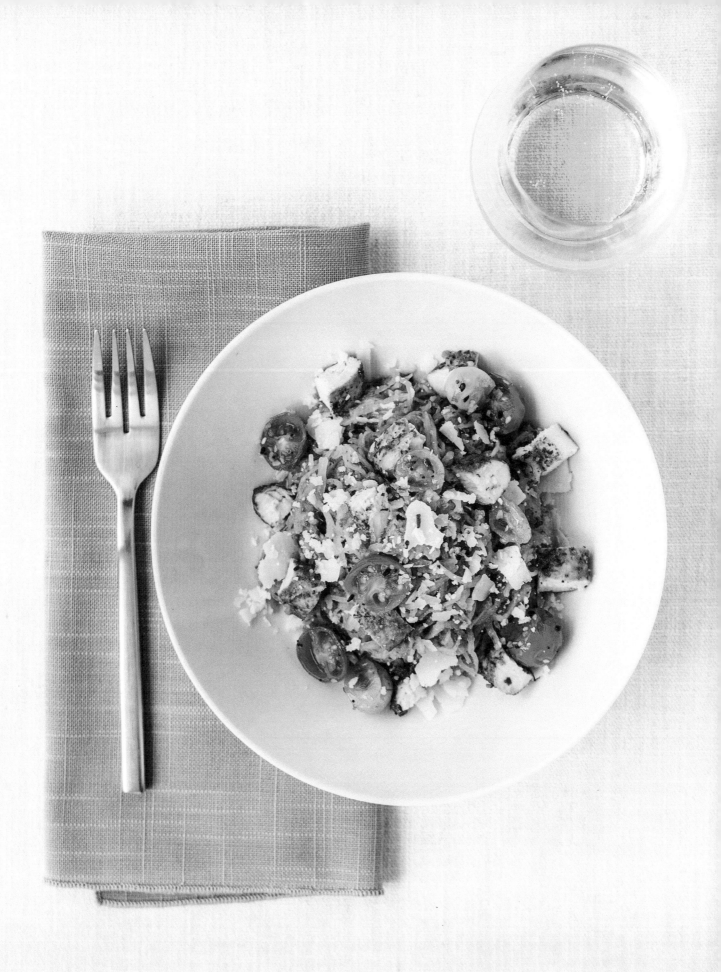

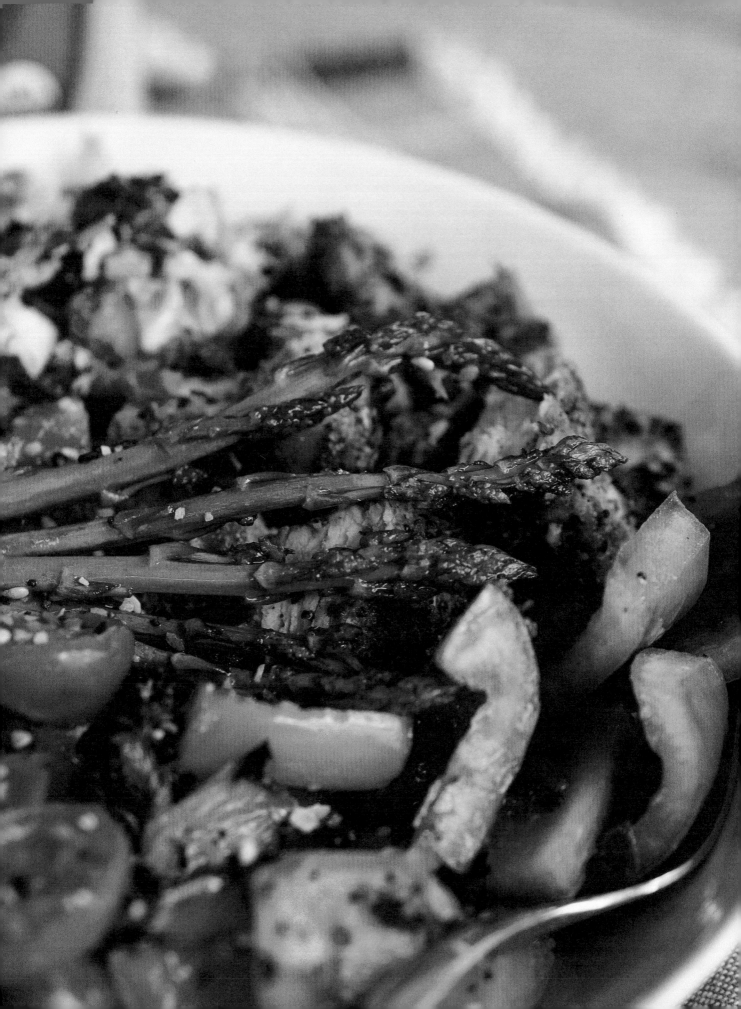

ROASTED VEGGIE BOWL

Clean out your produce drawer kids. These ain't your grandma's veggies.

Ingredients

Asparagus, trimmed

Brussels sprouts, shaved or halved

Broccoli florets

Bell pepper, sliced

Cauliflower rice

Grape or cherry tomatoes

Olive oil

Everything bagel seasoning

Chili lime seasoning

Feta cheese

Sriracha ranch dressing

Other Veggie Options:

Eggplant, peeled and cubed

Cauliflower florets

Zuchinni, diced

Directions

1. Preheat oven to 425°F and line a baking sheet with parchment paper.

2. On the baking sheet, make columns with each type of vegetable, cauliflower rice included.

3. Drizzle everything with olive oil and season veggies with bagel seasoning and chili lime, alternating seasoning between veggie columns.

4. Roast veggies until golden brown. 25 minutes typically gets the job done.

5. Build your bowl: top cauliflower rice with veggies, add crumbled feta and drizzle with Sriracha ranch. Get ready to please your palate!

Beth's Tip

In need of a protein boost? *Seersucker Chicken* (pg 16) is the perfect add on.

SHAVED BRUSSELS WITH BACON AND EGG

The tastiest way to elevate your brussels.

Ingredients

Brussels sprouts, shaved

Bacon

Olive oil

Everything bagel seasoning

Eggs

Feta cheese (optional)

Sriracha ranch dressing (optional)

Directions

1. Preheat oven to 425°F and line a baking sheet with parchment paper.

2. Add brussels sprouts to one half of the baking sheet. Drizzle with olive oil and season with bagel seasoning.

3. To the other half of the baking sheet, add however many bacon slices tickle your fancy.

4. Bake for 25 minutes, until brussels sprouts are roasted, and bacon is crispy.

5. Heat olive oil in a small skillet over medium-high heat. Crack an egg into the pan and cook to the desired level of doneness. I like the yolk to dress my brussels.

6. Build your bowl: fill your bowl with roasted brussels, top with crumbled bacon, and a fried egg. Be prepared to fall deep for the brussels.

Beth's Tip

If you're feeling extra fiesty, add some crumbled feta and a drizzle of Sriracha ranch.

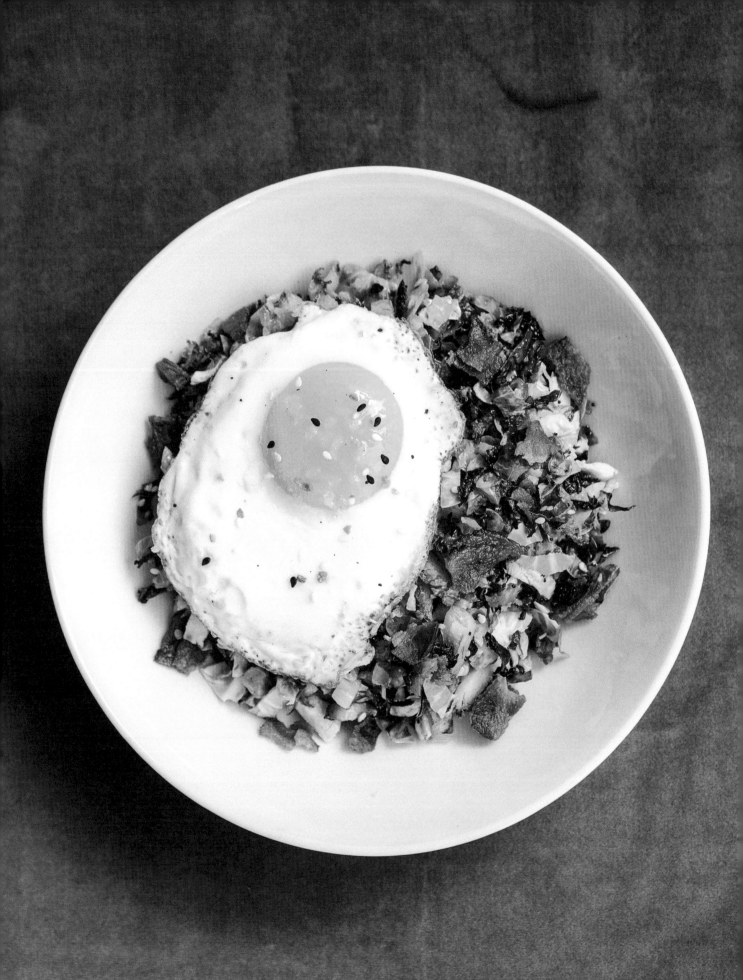

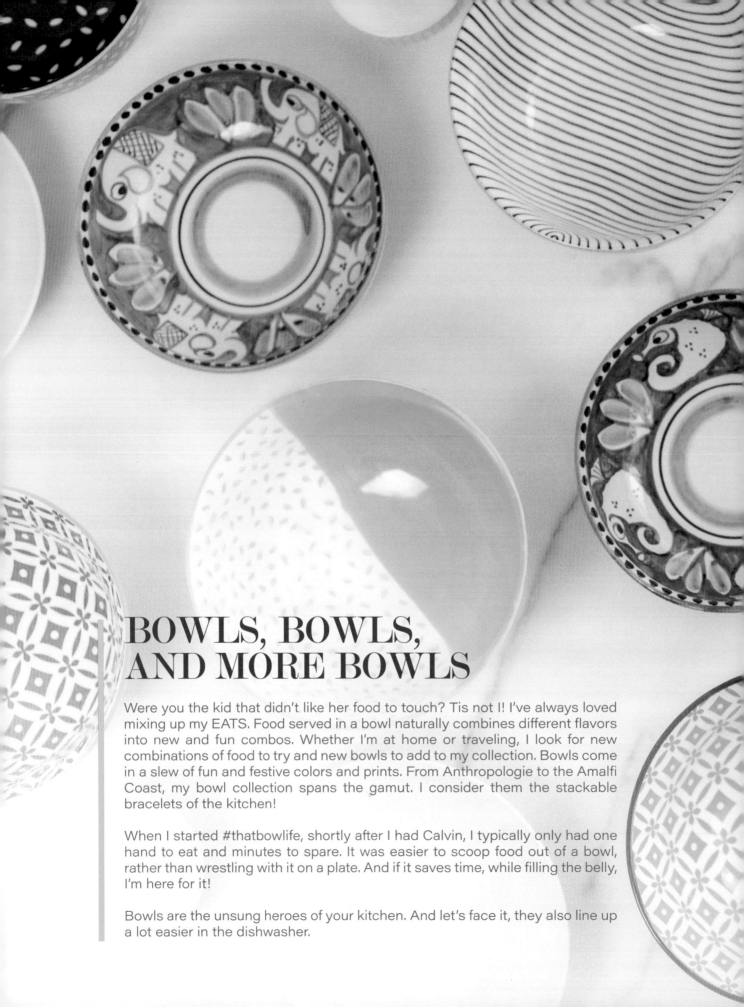

BOWLS, BOWLS, AND MORE BOWLS

Were you the kid that didn't like her food to touch? Tis not I! I've always loved mixing up my EATS. Food served in a bowl naturally combines different flavors into new and fun combos. Whether I'm at home or traveling, I look for new combinations of food to try and new bowls to add to my collection. Bowls come in a slew of fun and festive colors and prints. From Anthropologie to the Amalfi Coast, my bowl collection spans the gamut. I consider them the stackable bracelets of the kitchen!

When I started #thatbowlife, shortly after I had Calvin, I typically only had one hand to eat and minutes to spare. It was easier to scoop food out of a bowl, rather than wrestling with it on a plate. And if it saves time, while filling the belly, I'm here for it!

Bowls are the unsung heroes of your kitchen. And let's face it, they also line up a lot easier in the dishwasher.

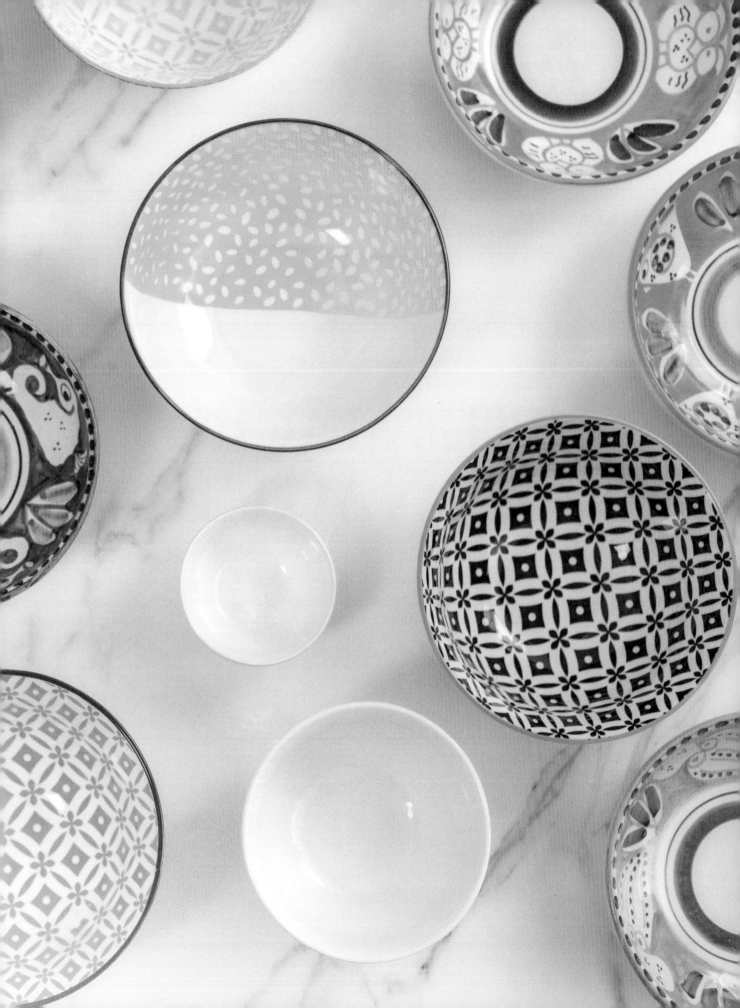

Chapter Two

THE MACRO MANAGER

Whether you're tracking macros or not,
these healthy eats will please all palates!

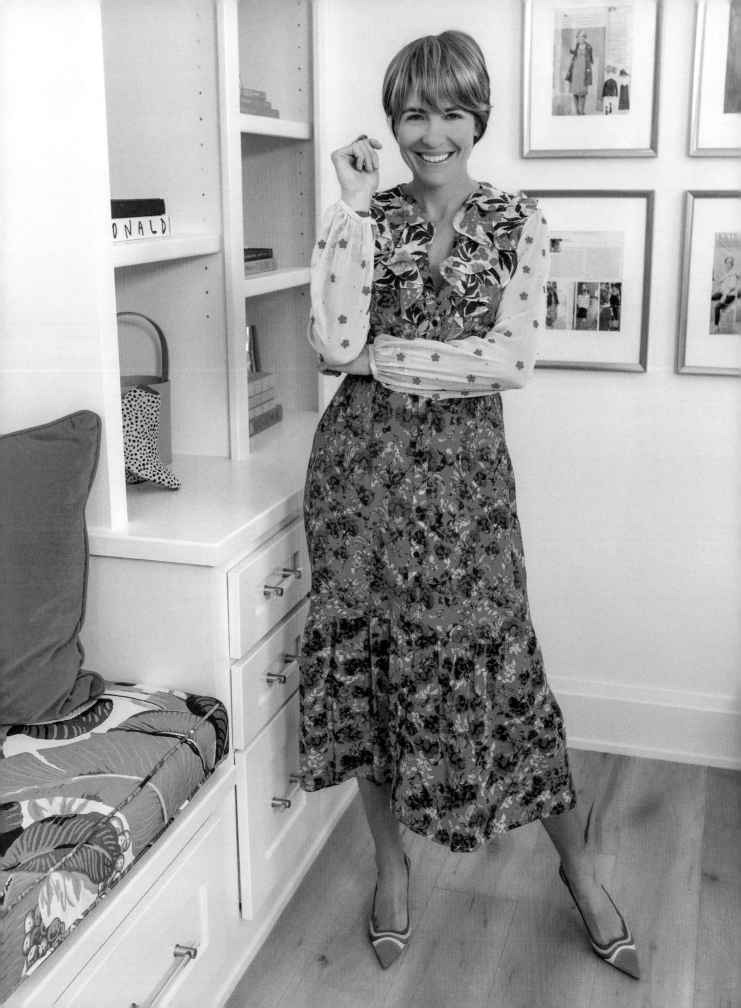

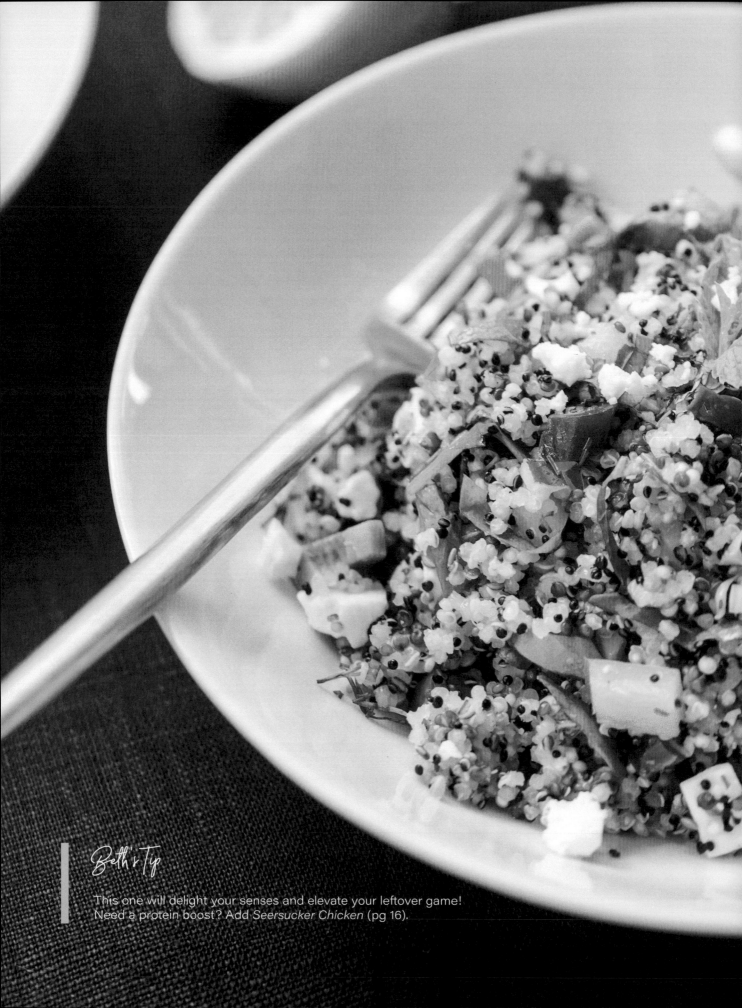

Beth's Tip

This one will delight your senses and elevate your leftover game!
Need a protein boost? Add *Seersucker Chicken* (pg 16).

GREEK QUINOA BOWL

Inspired by my dear friend in Lexington, chef Allison Davis. This one gets tastier as time goes on! Don't overthink it. Toss in what you have. Take out what you don't.

Ingredients

Quinoa

Yellow bell pepper— or any color bell pepper

Spinach

Mint

Dill

Dates

Red onion

Kalamata olives

Marinated artichokes

Feta cheese

Olive oil

Lemon juice

Salt and pepper

Directions

1. Cook quinoa according to package directions.

2. Chop all your veggies, herbs, dates, onion, olives, and artichokes.

3. Add quinoa to a large bowl and stir in the chopped salad ingredients, and feta.

   Rule of thumb: 2 cups of quinoa, 1 cup of veggies, and ¼ cup of everything else.

4. Drizzle everything with olive oil and the juice of 1-2 lemons.

5. Season with salt and pepper and get ready for love at first bite.

Beth's Tip

Dress up your burger by adding blue cheese, feta, or crumbled bacon to the burger mix.

CHILI LIME SEASONING BLEND

THE BLACK BEAN BURGER

This bad boy packs a protein punch. Even your beau won't know it's beefless.

Ingredients

2 cans of black beans

Chili lime seasoning

Olive oil

Bell pepper

Red onion

Zucchini

2 garlic cloves, minced

Quinoa

Worcestershire sauce

½ cup panko breadcrumbs

Eggs

Avocado

Directions

1. Preheat oven to 425°F and line a baking sheet with parchment paper.

2. Drain black beans and spread them on the baking sheet. Season with chili lime.

3. Roast beans for 10 minutes to dry them out a little bit. Don't suck out all the moisture, but you don't want a mushy burger.

4. While the beans are roasting, heat olive oil in a skillet over medium-high heat. Sauté ½ diced bell pepper, ½ diced red onion, diced zucchini, and garlic for about 5 minutes. Season with salt, pepper, and chili lime.

5. Cook quinoa according to package directions.

6. Gently blot cooked vegetables and quinoa with paper towels to remove excess moisture.

7. Place roasted black beans, 1-2 cups quinoa, and vegetables in a food processor with a few dashes of Worcestershire sauce, breadcrumbs, and 1 egg. Give it a good pulse until combined but not pureed.

8. Form mixture into 4 patties.

9. Using the same pan used for sautéing the veggies, cook patties for 3-5 minutes per side until crispy and golden brown.

10. Heat olive oil in a small skillet over medium-high heat. Crack an egg into the pan and cook to the desired level of doneness.

11. Build your burger: top burger patty with a fried egg and sliced avocado seasoned with chili lime. These pair beautifully with *All Day Everyday Arugula* (pg 19) or spinach. Who needs the beef?

CAULIFLOWER GNOCCHI WITH PESTO AND TOMATOES

Take it from this gnocchi lover: this one might surprise you.

Ingredients

Grape or cherry tomatoes

Everything bagel seasoning

Olive oil

Cauliflower gnocchi

Salt and pepper

Pesto

Parmesan cheese, shaved

Seersucker Chicken (pg 16)

Directions

1. Preheat oven to 400°F and line a baking sheet with parchment paper.

2. Spread the tomatoes onto the baking sheet. Drizzle with olive oil and season with bagel seasoning. Roast for 15-20 minutes.

3. While tomatoes are roasting, heat olive oil in a skillet over medium-high heat. Sauté cauliflower gnocchi until golden brown. **Do not add water** as the directions suggest. Season gnocchi with salt and pepper and add pesto.

4. Build your bowl: start with cauli pesto gnocchi and *Seersucker Chicken*. Top with roasted tomatoes and shaved parm. Devour until your tummy's content.

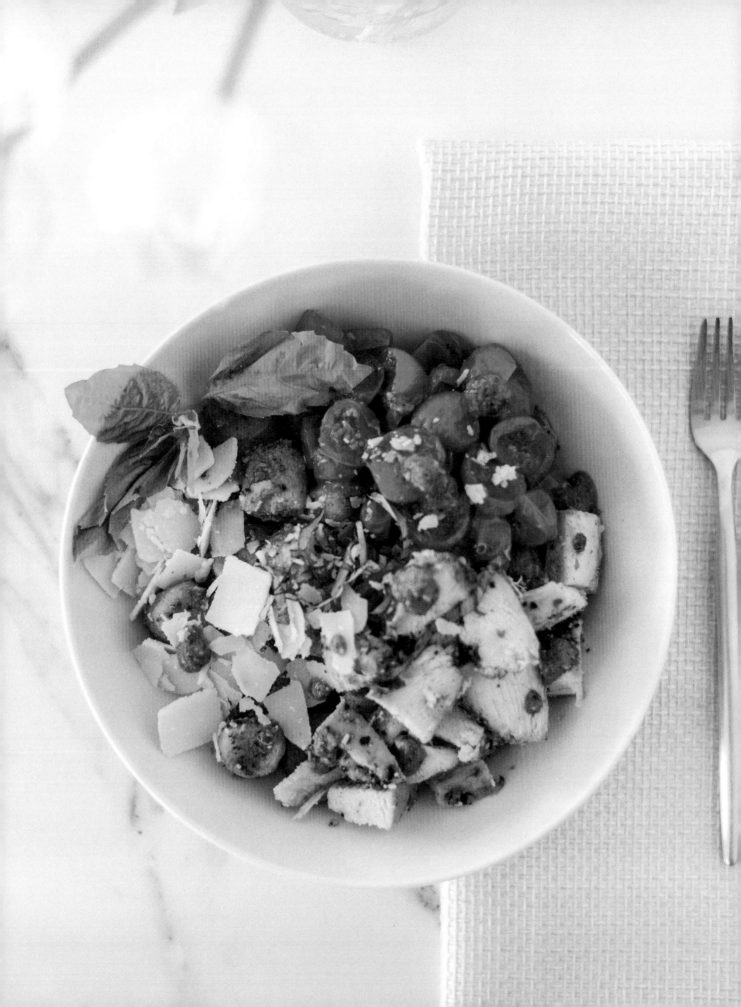

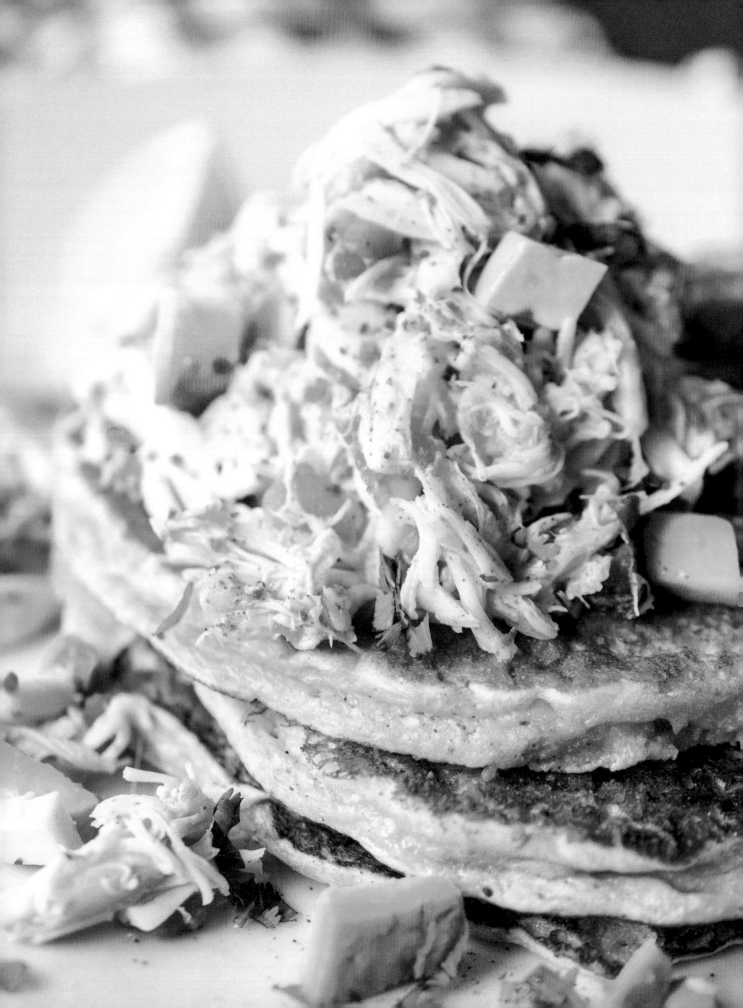

CRAB SALAD WITH PROTEIN CORN CAKES

This one takes the cake.

Ingredients

Crab Salad

Lump crab meat

Limes

Pico de gallo

Cilantro

Chili lime seasoning

Corn Cakes

Protein pancake mix

1 can organic creamed corn

Sugar

Coconut Oil

Avocado

Sriracha ranch dressing

Directions

Make the Crab Salad

1. Using your hands, break up crabmeat and toss it into a bowl.

2. Add the juice of 1-2 limes, a few spoonfuls of pico de gallo, and a palmful of chopped cilantro. Season with chili lime.

3. Refrigerate until ready to use.

Make the Corn Cakes

1. Follow the package instructions to make protein pancakes, replacing the liquid with 1 can of creamed corn. Add a couple pinches of sugar. Mix until combined.

2. Heat coconut oil in a large skillet or on a griddle over medium-high heat.

3. Drop corn cake batter onto hot griddle and cook until edges are golden crispy and the middle is fluffy. Flipping halfway through.

4. Dress your cake with crab salad, top with diced avocado, and a drizzle of Sriracha ranch. Eat your heart out.

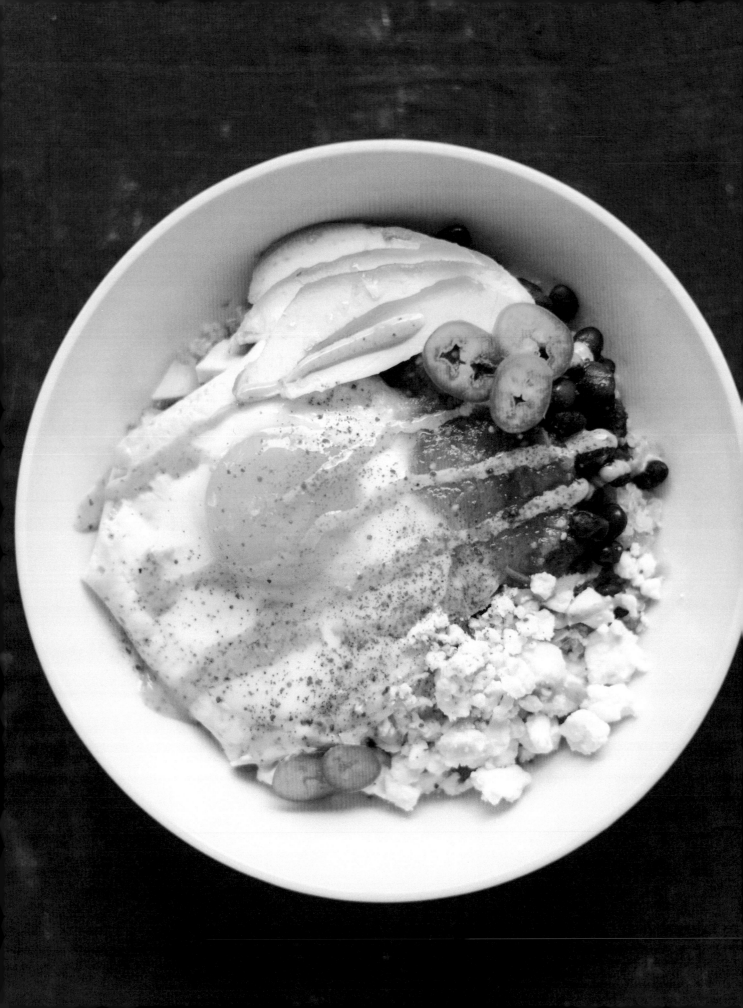

THE ELEVATED EGG BOWL

Inspired by one of my favorite restaurants in Indy. This is quite possibly the best regular macro meal.

Ingredients

Quinoa

Black beans

Chili lime seasoning

Eggs

Avocado

Feta cheese

Salsa verde

Sriracha ranch dressing

Directions

1. Cook quinoa according to package directions.

2. In a small saucepan, heat black beans and season with chili lime.

3. Heat olive oil in a small skillet over medium-high heat. Crack an egg into the pan and cook until the desired level of doneness—I like my yolk to dress my bowl.

4. Build your bowl: layer quinoa and black beans. Add your fried egg. Top with diced avocado, feta, salsa verde, and a drizzle of Sriracha ranch. You're welcome!

ONE PAN SAUSAGE

Minimal dishes. Maximum flavor.

Ingredients

Chicken sausage

Fuji apples

Sweet potatoes

Broccoli

Brussels sprouts

Olive oil

Cinnamon

Chili lime seasoning

Stone ground mustard (optional)

Directions

1. Preheat oven to 425°F and line a baking sheet with parchment paper.

2. Cut chicken sausage into thick slices. Chop apples, sweet potatoes, and veggies into bite-size pieces.

3. Make three columns on your baking sheet: one of chicken sausage, one of apples and sweet potatoes, and one of broccoli and brussels.

4. Drizzle everything with olive oil. Season apples and sweet potatoes with cinnamon. Season broccoli and brussels with chili lime.

5. Roast for 25 minutes until golden brown.

6. Build your bowl: mix it all up, top with mustard, and put it in a bowl and enjoy not having dish duty.

Beth's Tip

Any and every veggie will work in this recipe.
Cauliflower, bell peppers, asparagus... the list goes on.
Use what you have!

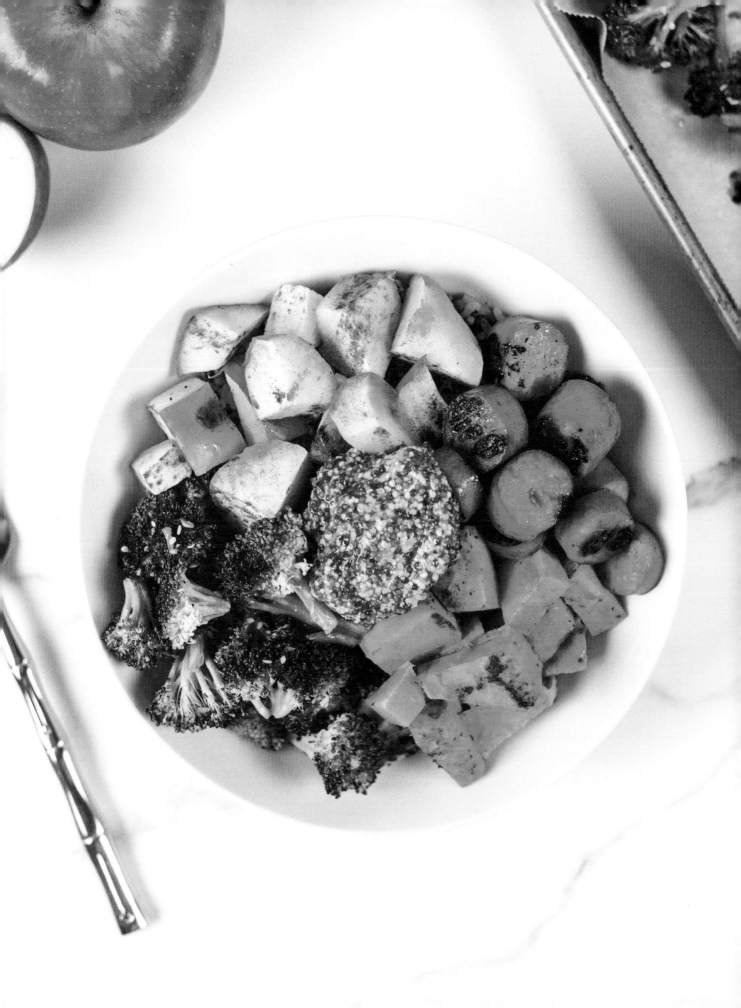

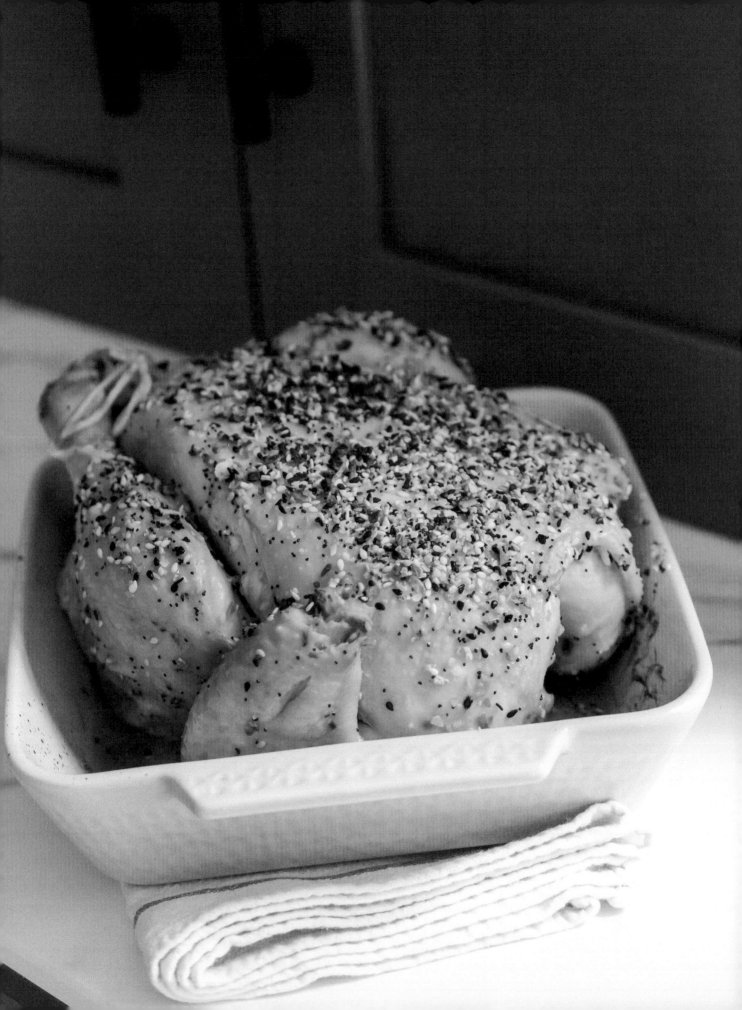

NONNIE'S ROASTED CHICKEN
WITH GREEN BEANS AND SWEET POTATO MASH

Don't let this one intimidate you.
This is one of the first meals Nonnie ever taught me to make. Easy breezy.

Ingredients

Roasted Chicken

Whole chicken

Olive oil

Seasoning of choice:
everything bagel seasoning,
lemon pepper, or chili lime
seasoning

Lemon

Green Beans

Bacon

Green beans, canned or fresh

Apple cider vinegar

Sweet Potato Mash

Sweet potatoes

Ghee or butter

Cinnamon

Directions

Roasted Chicken

1. Preheat oven to 350°F.

2. Get frisky with your chicken. Check the cavity and remove the packet of innards. Give the bird a good rinse inside and out and then pat dry, inside and out, with paper towels.

3. Massage the chicken with olive oil and then heavily coat the exterior with a seasoning of choice.

4. Chop the lemon into a few big pieces and stuff those inside the cavity.

5. Place chicken in a shallow roasting pan, breast-side up, tucking the wing tips under so they don't burn. Roast chicken for about 20 minutes per pound.

On to the green beans and sweet potatoes—this is the easy part.

Green Beans

1. When the chicken has 15-20 minutes left, start working on the green beans.

2. Line a microwave-safe plate with paper towels. Place bacon slices on the plate without overlapping. Microwave bacon for 3-4 minutes until extra crispy. Pat dry and crumble.

3. Heat olive oil in a skillet over medium-high heat. Drain canned green beans and add them to the skillet. Season beans with the same seasoning used on the chicken and heat until warmed through, approximately 5 minutes.

4. Add 2-3 capfuls of apple cider vinegar to the green beans and stir in the crumbled bacon.

Continued on next page.

Directions

Sweet Potato Mash

1. Scrub the sweet potatoes and pat them dry. Stab each potato several times with a fork.

2. Rub potatoes with olive oil and place on a microwave-safe plate. Microwave on high for 5-10 minutes, until soft.

3. Slice potatoes in half and mash with a generous amount of ghee and a dash of cinnamon.

4. Build you bowl: line the base of your bowl with sweet potato mash. Dress with sliced chicken and green beans and enjoy this healthy, downhome meal. #nonnieapproved

Beth's Tip

I prefer canned green beans for this recipe and, if you're in a time crunch, don't hesitate to get a rotisserie chicken. #convenience

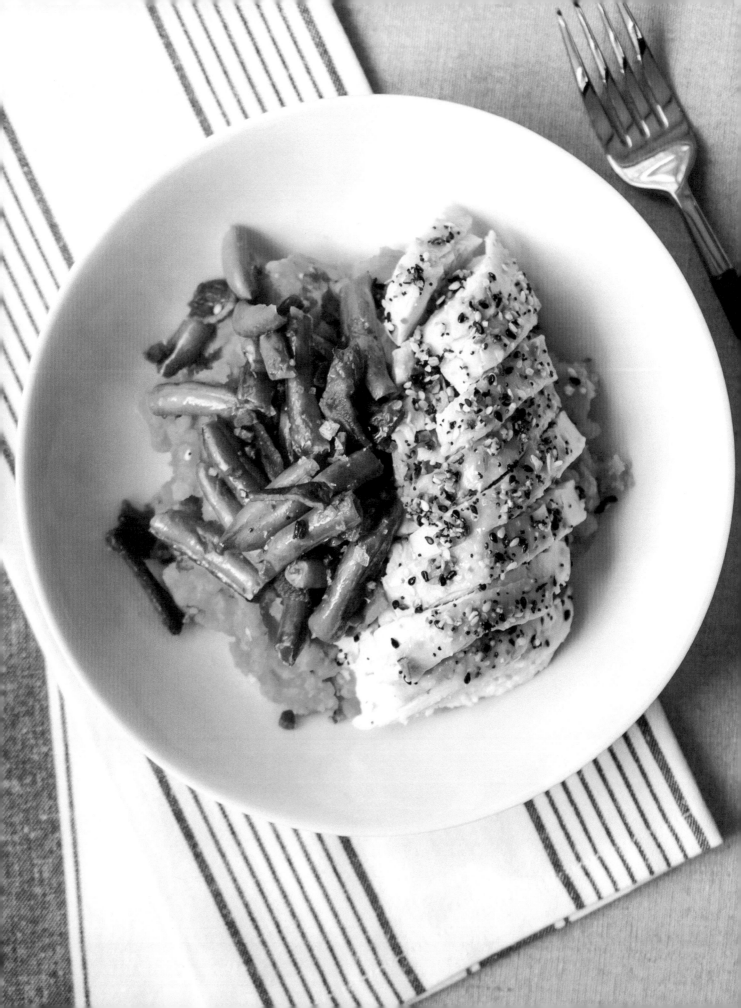

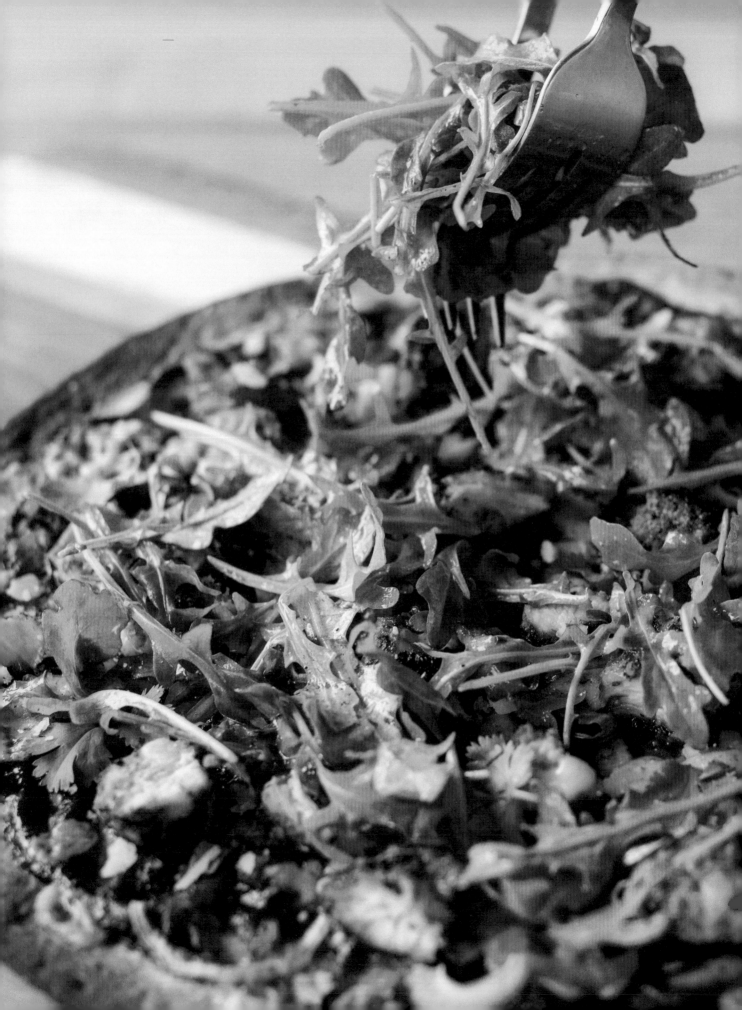

BARBECUE CHICKEN PIZZA

This one rivals the real deal.

Ingredients

Cauliflower pizza crust

Olive oil

Barbecue sauce

Red onion

Cilantro

Parmesan cheese, finely grated

Seersucker Chicken (pg 16)

All Day Every Day Arugula
(pg 19)

Directions

1. Preheat oven to 350°F.

2. Brush the cauliflower pizza crust with olive oil and place DIRECTLY onto the oven rack for about 5 minutes shy of the package directions.

3. Remove the crust from the oven, but very gently, she's fragile. Spread a layer of BBQ sauce onto the crust and top with chopped *Seersucker Chicken*, sliced red onion, chopped cilantro, and parm.

4. Put pizza back in the oven just long enough to melt the cheese.

5. Top with *All Day Everyday Arugula* either on top or on the side. Get after it!

MEXI BOWL

This meal ignited my love affair with bowls!

Ingredients

Seersucker Chicken (pg 16)

Olive oil

Cauliflower rice

Bell pepper

Chili lime seasoning

Feta cheese

Greek yogurt

Avocado

Jalapeño

Salsa verde

Directions

1. Make *Seersucker Chicken.*

2. While chicken bakes, heat olive oil in a skillet over medium-high heat.

3. Sauté cauliflower rice and chopped bell pepper for 5-7 minutes. Season generously with chili lime.

4. Build your bowl: fill bowl with the cauliflower rice and chopped pepper mixture. Top with sliced *Seersucker Chicken.*

5. Top with crumbled feta, a dollop of greek yogurt, diced avocado seasoned with chili lime, sliced jalapeño, and salsa verde. Be prepared to be a B O W L I E V E R!

Beth's Tip

If you're not low-carbing, add black beans, corn, quinoa or roasted sweet potatoes.

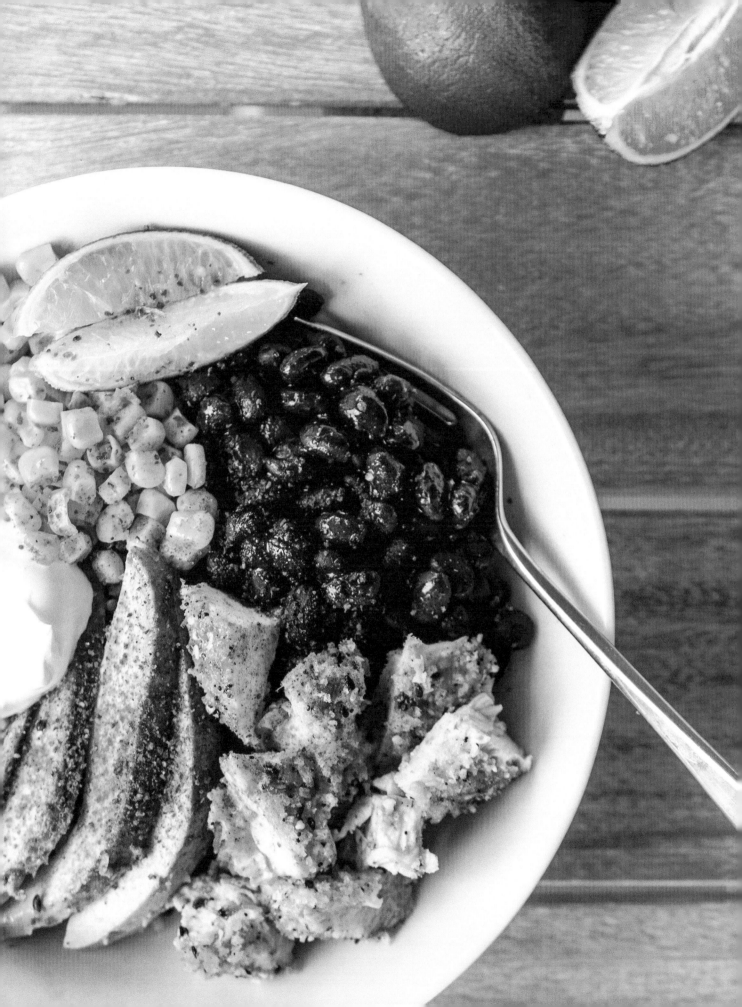

SEERSUCKER CHICKEN AND WAFFLES

This favorite southern fare comes from my treasured time in Kentucky. It's so freakin' simple, it's silly.

Ingredients

Seersucker Chicken (pg 16)

Protein waffle mix

Cinnamon

Vanilla

Coconut oil

Maple syrup

Directions

1. Make Seersucker Chicken.

2. While chicken bakes, prepare waffle mix according to package directions.

3. Add 3 or 4 dashes of cinnamon and a splash of vanilla to the waffle batter.

4. Grease waffle iron with coconut oil and cook waffles until golden brown.

5. Top waffles with Seersucker Chicken and warm maple syrup. Hey there, breakfast for dinner!

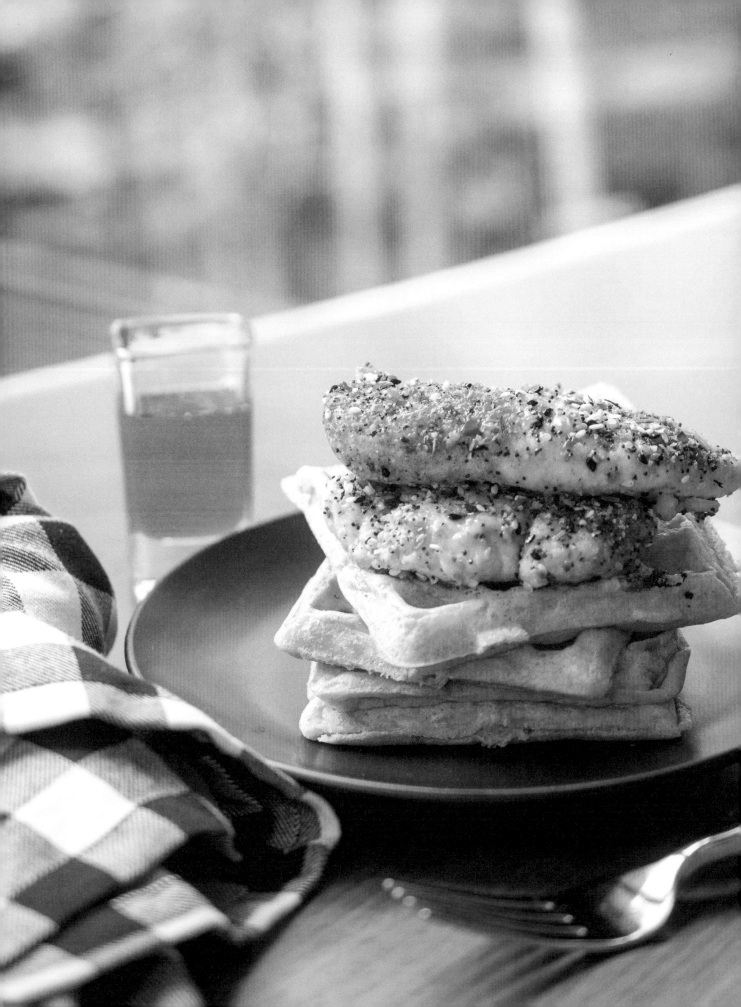

PEANUT BUTTER APPLES AND BRIE

Just like a grilled cheese, but fancy.

Ingredients

Cinnamon raisin bread

Coconut oil

Cinnamon

Peanut butter

Jam or preserves

Apples

Brie

Directions

1. Spread coconut oil on the outside of two slices of cinnamon raisin bread and sprinkle with cinnamon.

2. Spread peanut butter on one slice of bread and jam on the other slice of bread.

3. Top peanut butter slice with a layer of thinly sliced apples and brie. Put the two slices of bread together to form a sandwich.

4. Heat a large skillet or griddle over medium-high heat and cook sammy until both sides are golden brown. Slice and serve.

Beth's Tip

Pairs nicely with *All Day Everyday Arugula* (pg 19)—as does everything else!

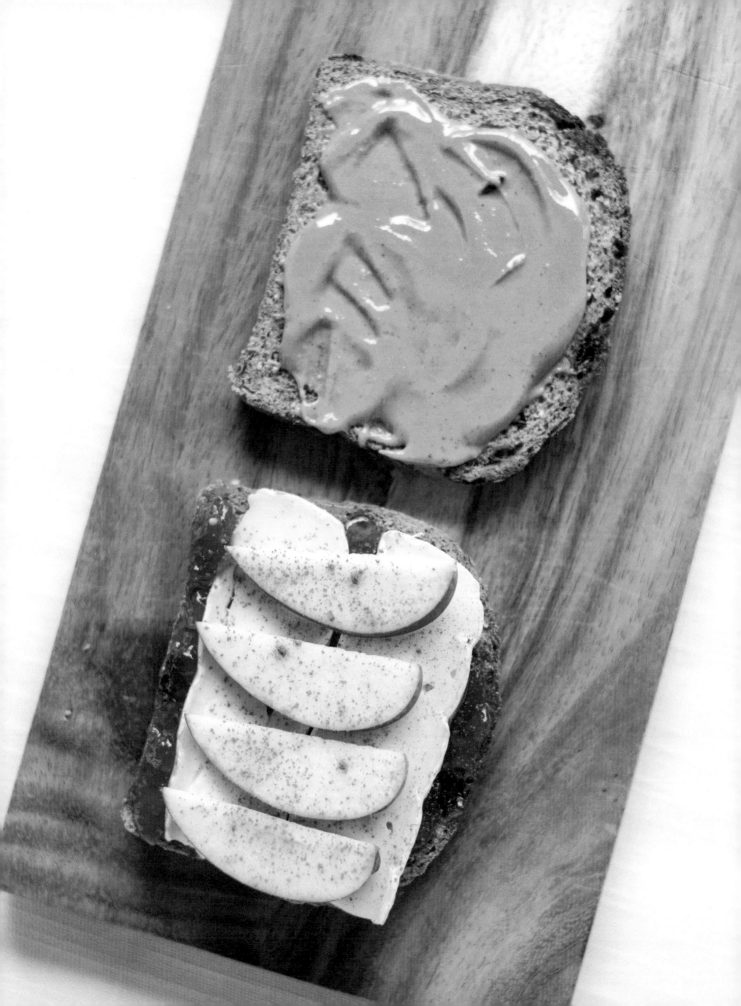

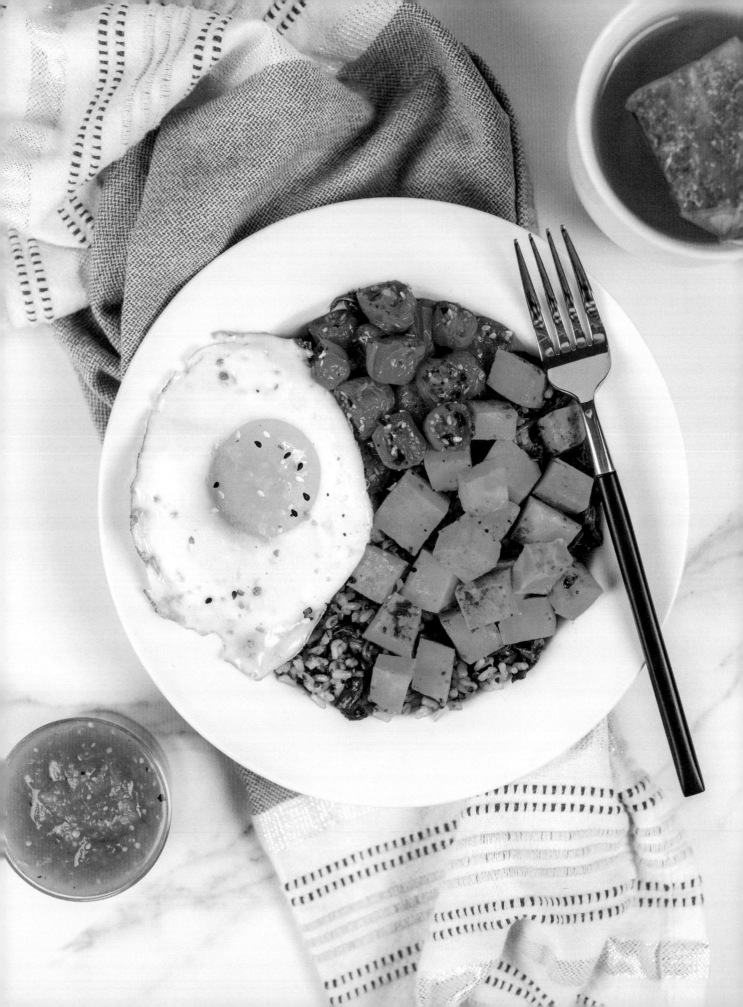

THE BRECK BOWL

Inspired by one of my fave breakfast spots in Breckenridge, CO.
This one is tasty morning, noon, and night.

Ingredients

Sweet potatoes

Grape or cherry tomatoes

Cinnamon

Everything bagel seasoning

Quinoa

Olive oil

Baby spinach

Lemon

Egg

Salsa verde

Directions

1. Preheat oven to 425°F and line a baking sheet with parchment paper.

2. Peel and cube sweet potatoes and cut tomatoes in half.

3. Add sweet potatoes to one half of the baking sheet and tomatoes to the other half. Drizzle everything with olive oil. Season potatoes with cinnamon and season tomatoes with bagel seasoning. Bake for 25 minutes.

4. Cook quinoa according to package directions.

5. Heat olive oil in a large skillet over medium-high heat. Add a couple of handfuls of baby spinach and sauté until wilted. Transfer spinach to a plate and add a squeeze of lemon juice.

6. Using the same skillet, fry an egg to the desired level of doneness.

7. Build your bowl: start with a base of quinoa and add roasted veggies. Top with a fried egg, garnish with salsa verde, and enjoy all times of the day.

NONNIE'S TOMATO BASIL PASTA

A dish I've loved ever since I was little, and I'm certain you will too.

Ingredients

Angel hair or penne pasta — preferrably gluten free

Olive oil

2 cloves garlic, minced

2 (14 oz) cans organic petite-diced tomatoes

Salt and pepper

Italian seasoning

Baby spinach

Basil

Parmesan cheese, shaved

Directions

1. Bring a large pot of salted water to a boil and cook pasta according to package directions.

2. Heat olive oil in a large sauté pan over medium-high heat. Sauté minced garlic for a quick minute, then add diced tomatoes with their juice.

3. Season the sauce with salt, pepper, and Italian seasoning. Lower heat and simmer until sauce is reduced slightly.

4. Drain pasta and add to the sauce in the sauté pan, toss to coat.

5. Add a couple of handfuls of baby spinach to the hot pasta and stir until wilted.

6. Build your bowl: garnish bowls of pasta with fresh basil and shaved parm. Add a glass of white wine and bon appétit.

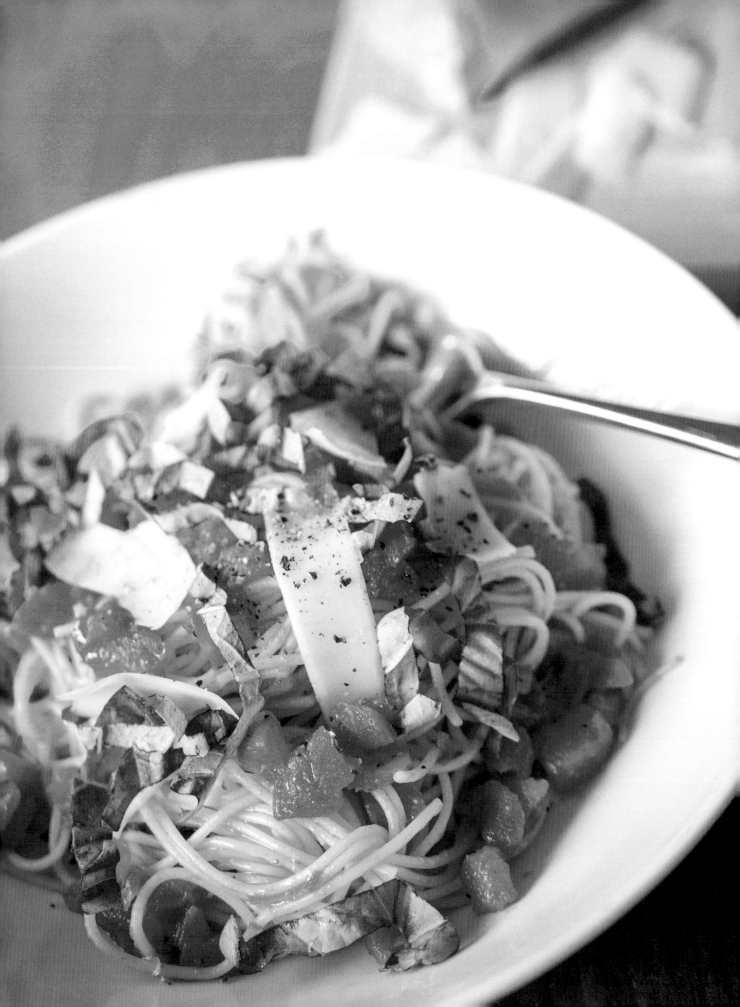

CHICKEN PICCATA

One of my fam's faves. I suspect it might become one of yours too.

Ingredients

Boneless, skinless chicken breasts or tenderloins

Italian seasoned panko breadcrumbs

Parmesan cheese, finely grated

Everything bagel seasoning

Salt and pepper

Avocado oil

1 tablespoon butter

½ cup chicken broth

¼ cup white wine

Lemon

Capers

Pasta, for serving — preferably gluten free

Directions

1. Make chicken breading by combining healthy palmfuls of italian panko and parm, and a good dash of bagel seasoning.

2. Season chicken with salt and pepper and coat both sides with the breading mixture.

3. Heat avocado oil in a large skillet over medium-high heat. Add chicken and cook 4-5 minutes on each side, until cooked through.

4. Transfer chicken to a plate.

5. To the same skillet, add butter, chicken broth, white wine, juice of half a lemon, and capers. Bring sauce to boil, scraping up the brown bits on the bottom of the pan for all the extra-yummy flavor. Turn heat down and simmer until slightly reduced.

6. Transfer the chicken back to the sauce and turn to coat.

7. If you're low-carbing this, serve chicken with *All Day Everyday Arugula* (pg 19) and roasted broccoli. If you've got carbs to spare, serve with gluten free pasta. This one is a crowd-pleaser with the entire Chappo crew.

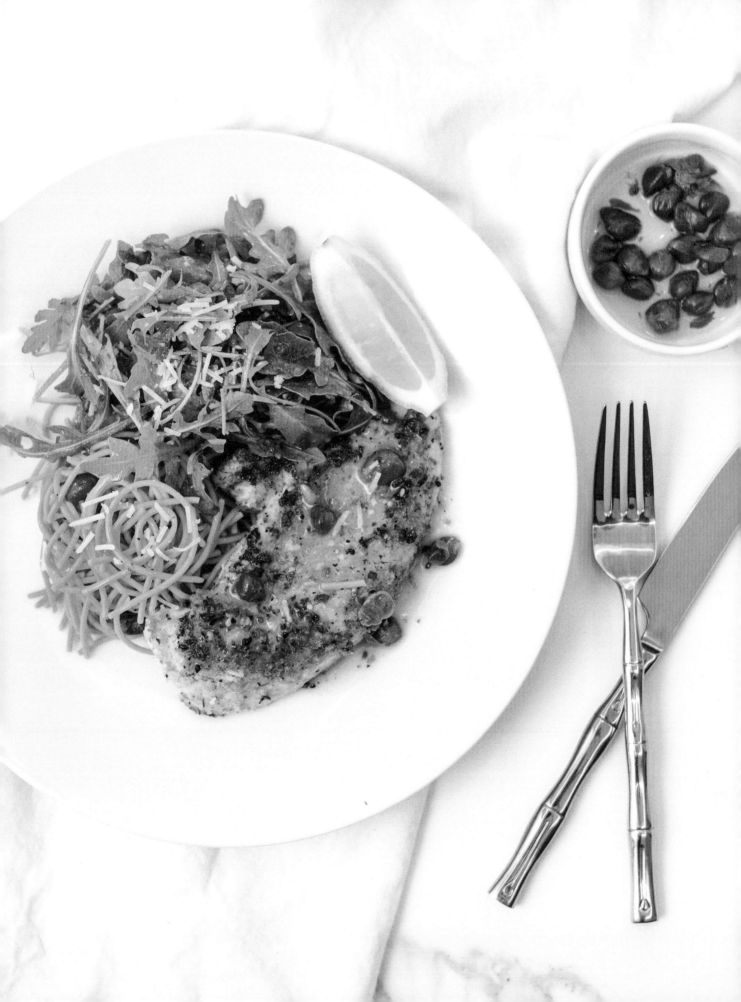

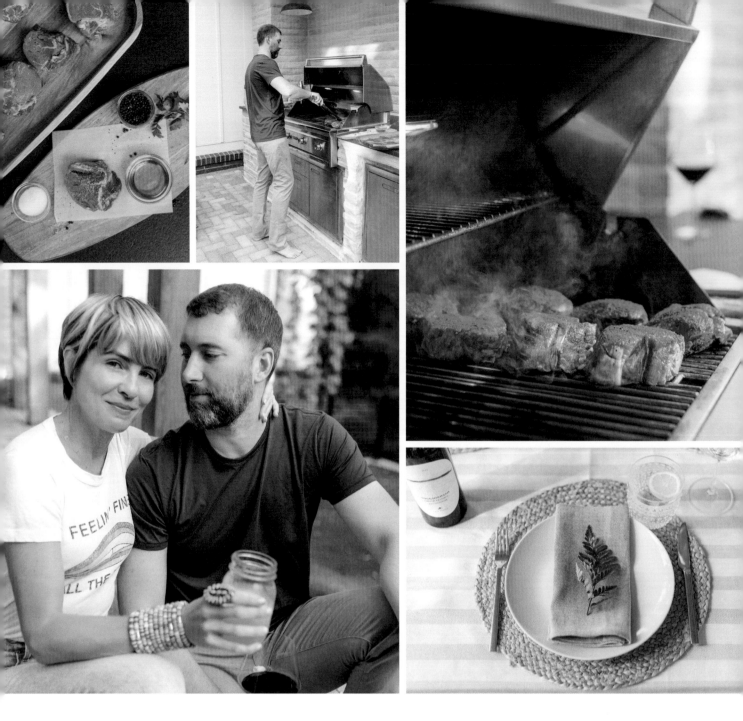

JOHNNY'S FILETS

If you've ever had dinner at the Chappo household, you've probably had Johnny's filets. They're a home run. They're easy. They're a crowd-pleaser. And the chef, a.k.a. Johnny, takes such pride in his cooking techniques. It always starts with Johnny taking a trip to Costco, where he, in pure Johnny form, over analyzes the meat section to find the perfect filets. Once I made the Costco run for the steaks, and he claimed my "picker was off." So, alas, we leave that job to him.

Johnny has this meal down to a science and whether we're celebrating a birthday, achievement, hosting a family gathering, or having a dinner party; this is pretty much our meal of choice. But beware, while the kids and I joke that this is our favorite meal, it comes at a cost. And by cost, we mean having to hear the chef brag about his searing and seasoning techniques. How each steak is better than the last one he cooked. How the flavor is unmatched by famous steakhouses. I mean, It. Never. Fails. But you know what, he's kinda spot on.

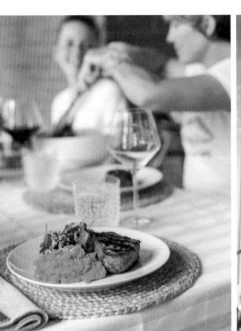
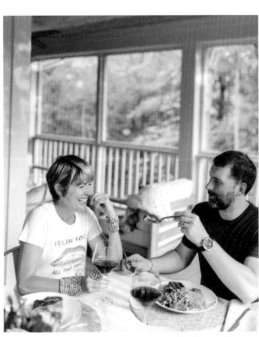
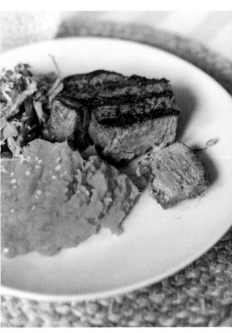

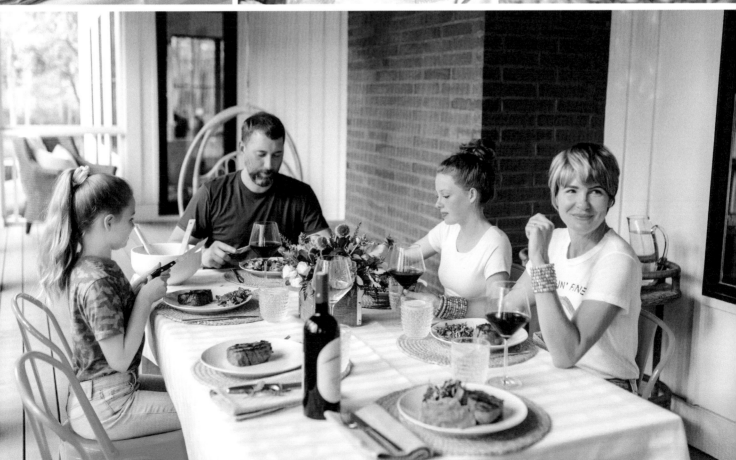

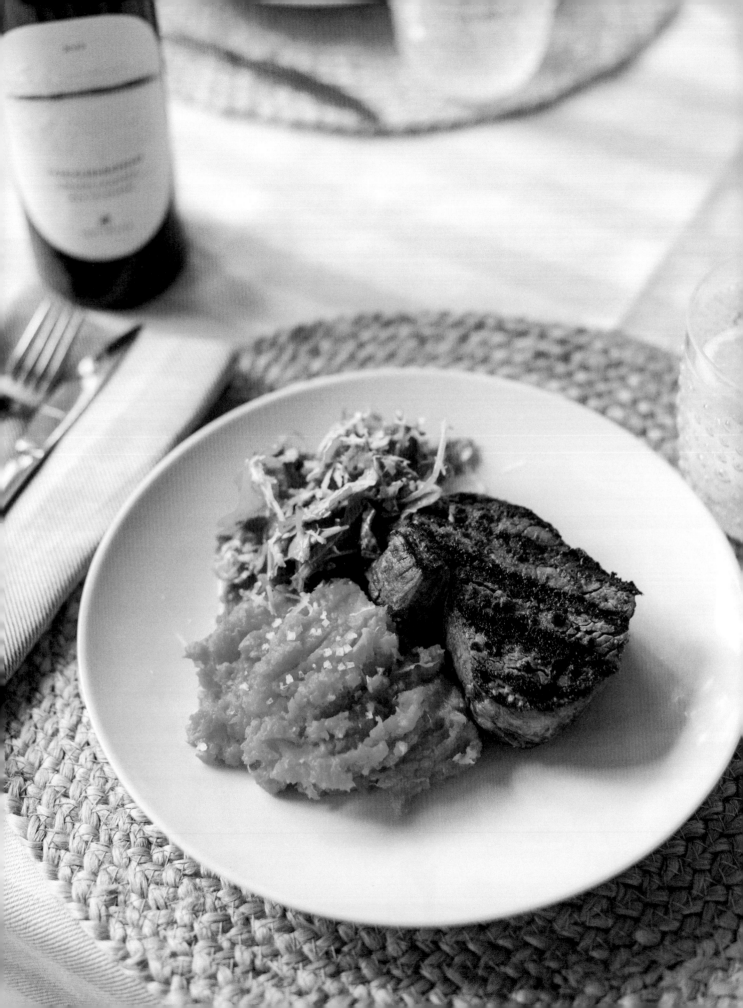

JOHNNY'S FILETS

Ingredients

Filet mignon, thick cut (2-2.5 inches)

Paprika

Sea salt

Cracked pepper

Avocado oil

Directions

On the Grill

1. Remove filets from the fridge and let sit at room temp for 20-30 minutes.

2. Preheat grill to 500°F.

3. Season steaks heavily on both sides with paprika, salt, and pepper.

4. Sear steak over open flame, or high heat, for 3 minutes per side.

5. Turn off one grill burner, move steaks to the lower heat side of the grill, and close the lid.

6. Keep grill closed and allow steaks to cook for another 3 minutes, or until they reach the desired temperature. Medium-rare steaks should be soft to the touch.

In the Oven

1. Remove filets from the fridge and let sit at room temp for 20-30 minutes.

2. Preheat oven to 450°F.

3. Season steaks heavily on both sides with paprika, salt, and pepper.

4. In an oven-safe skillet, heat oil over medium-high heat. Once oil is nice and hot, sear the steaks for 3 minutes per side.

5. Once seared, transfer the entire pan to preheated oven for 3-5 minutes, or until steaks reach the desired temperature. We like medium-rare, so we do about 3 minutes in the oven.

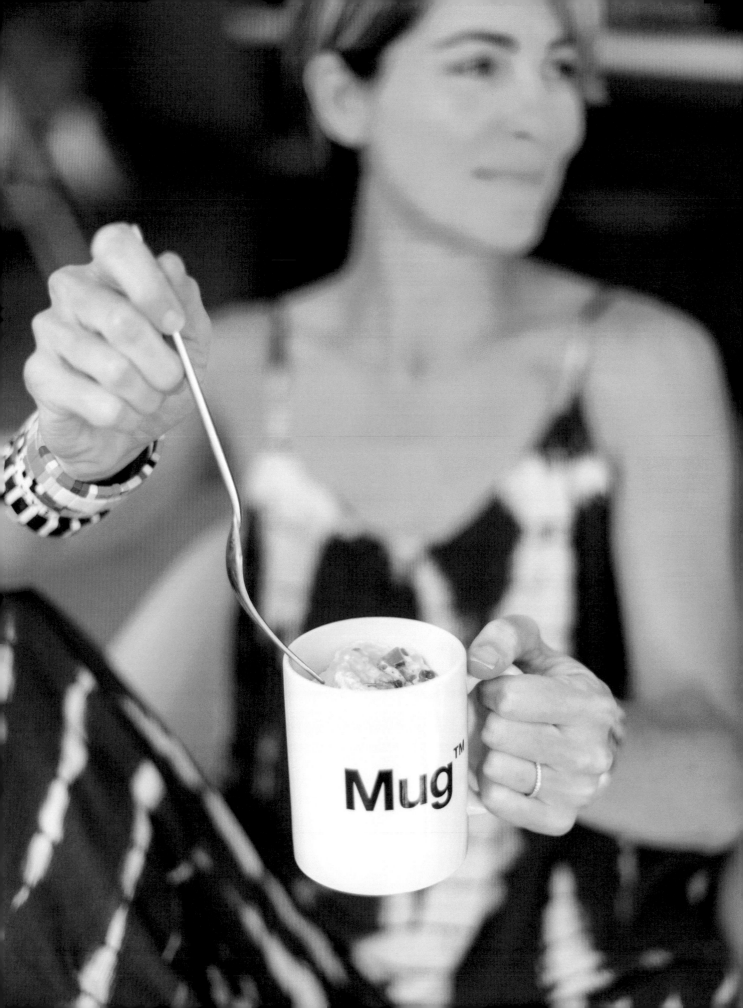

Chapter Three

SNACK ATTACK

Ever in a pinch?
Rest assured, these easy eats will get the job done!

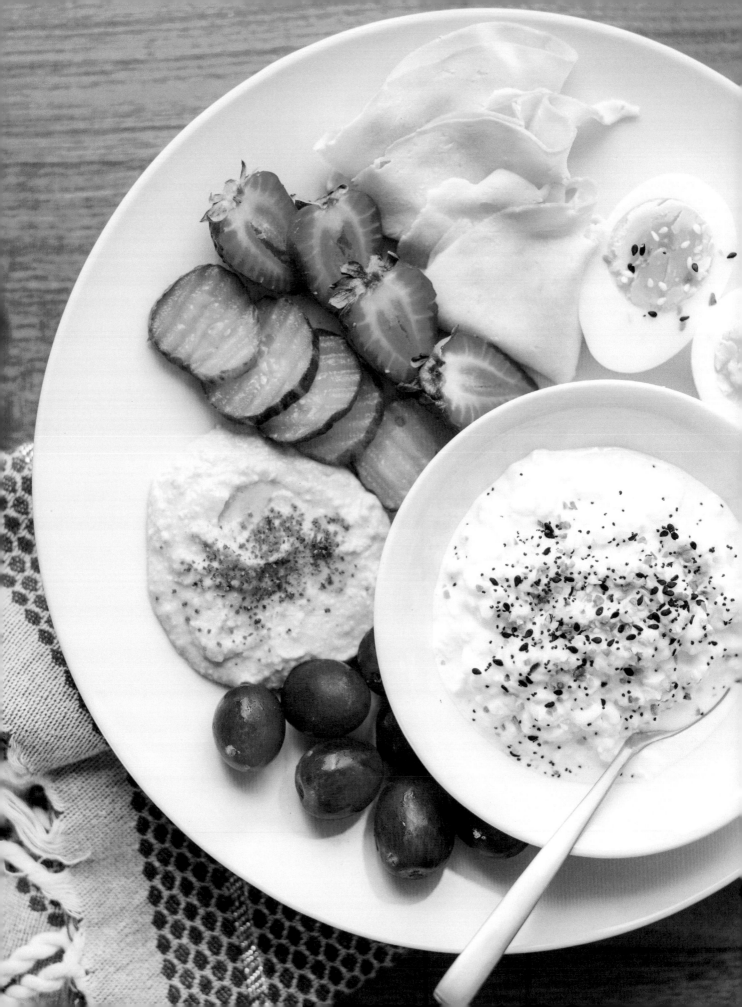

SNACKY PLATE

There are no rules. This is how I play with my snacks.

Ingredients

Hummus

Deli turkey

Hard-boiled eggs

Everything bagel seasoning

Chili lime seasoning

Strawberries

Grapes

Pickles

Cottage cheese

Other options:

Sliced avocado with salsa

Apples with peanut butter

Veggies

Olives

Directions

1. Spread hummus onto sliced turkey and roll up.

2. Slice hard-boiled eggs and season with bagel seasoning.

3. Cut strawberries in half and use grapes as they are.

4. Add a dollop of hummus, season with chili lime.

5. Add a few pickle slices.

6. Top a scoop of cottage cheese with bagel seasoning.

7. Arrange all your snack items on a nice big plate and nosh away!

EGG MUFFINS

Like a bowl, no rules needed. Add what you wish.

Ingredients

Coconut oil, for the muffin tin

12 eggs

Milk

Prosciutto

Bell pepper

Spinach

Cheddar cheese, shredded

Directions

1. Preheat oven to 350°F and grease a 12-cup muffin tin with coconut oil.

2. Crack eggs into a large bowl, add a splash of milk, and beat until light and fluffy.

3. Add diced pepper, chopped prosciutto, chopped spinach, and shredded cheddar.

4. Pour the mixture evenly into the muffin tin, filling muffin cups to the top.

5. Bake for 15-20 minutes until eggs are set. You can test with a toothpick to see if the eggs are firm and cooked through. LEFTOVERS? Hang on to 'em for tomorrow's breakfast.

Beth's Tip

Toss these on a *Snacky Plate* (pg 85).

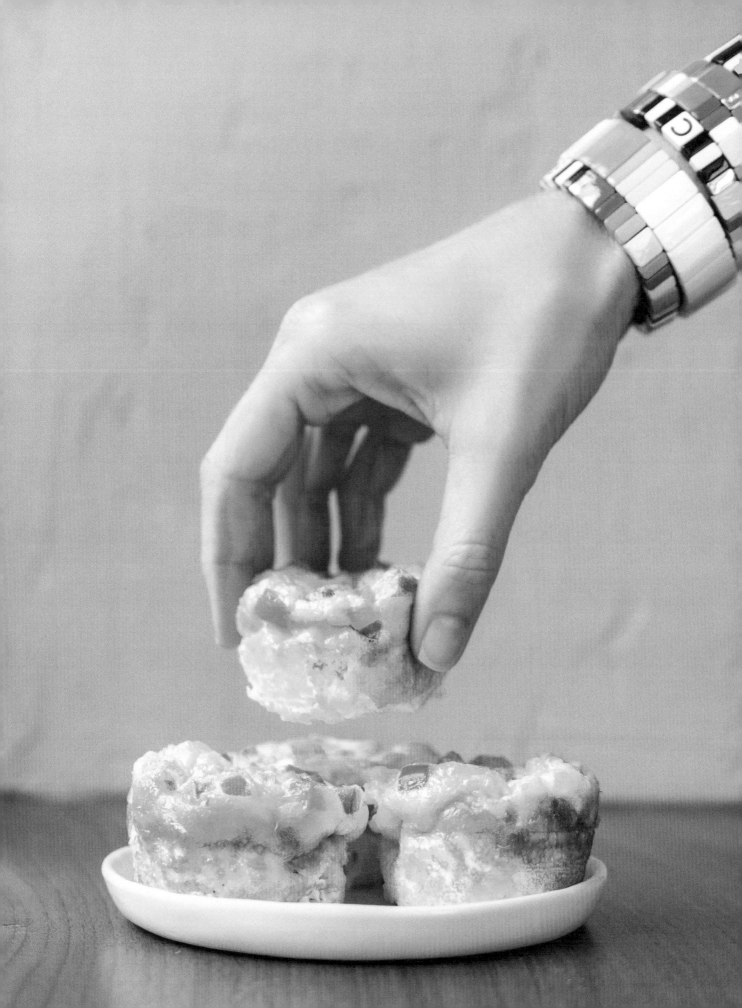

SPINACH PROTEIN MUFFINS

What's better than tricking your kids into eating healthy?!

Ingredients

Coconut oil, for the muffin tin

Protein pancake mix

Banana

Spinach

Cinnamon

Mini chocolate chips

Directions

1. Preheat oven to 350°F and grease a mini muffin tin with coconut oil.

2. To a blender, add pancake mix and liquid, according to the package directions for one batch of batter.

3. Add 1 banana, a handful of spinach and a dash of cinnamon. Blend until smooth.

4. Pour the batter into prepared muffin cups and top each muffin with mini chocolate chips.

5. Bake muffins for 15 minutes, until edges are golden brown. Beware, if you're like me, one of these is simply not enough!

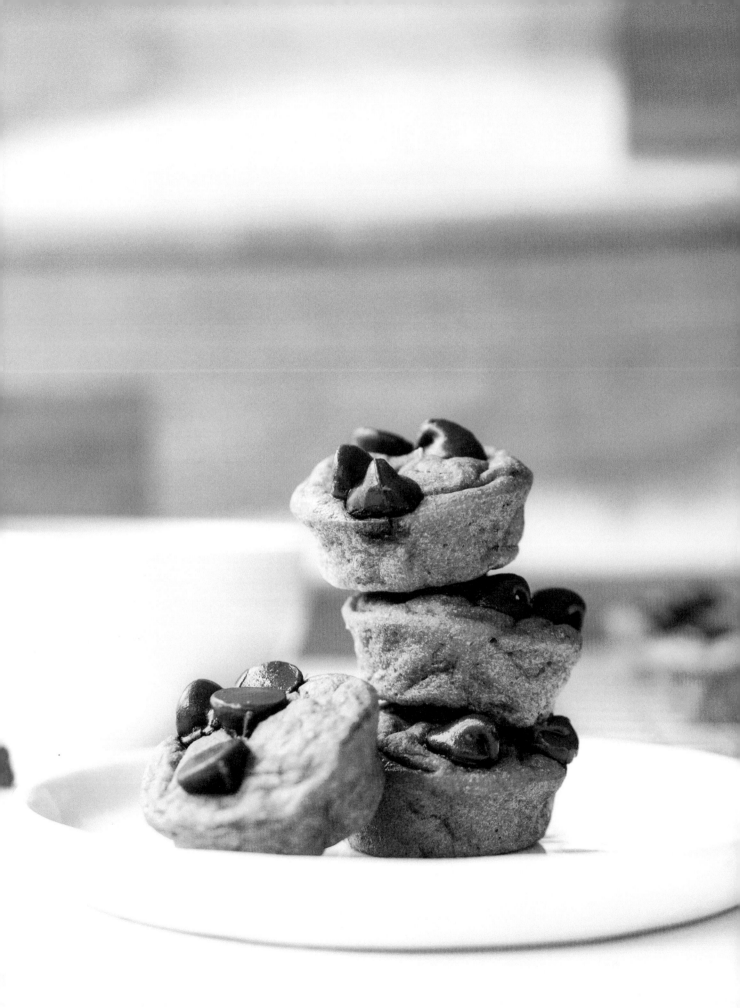

ACAI-LESS ACAI BOWL

Get your phone ready. These bowls are Insta worthy!

Ingredients

Frozen fruit

Banana

Berries—strawberries, blueberries, raspberries

Granola

Unsweetened shredded coconut

Peanut butter or nut butter

Directions

1. To a blender, add frozen fruit and a smidge of water. Blend just long enough to puree the fruit. The mixture should be thick.

2. Build your bowl: add blended fruit to the bottom of a bowl. Layer the top with pretty rows of sliced banana, berries, granola, coconut and a spoonful of peanut butter.

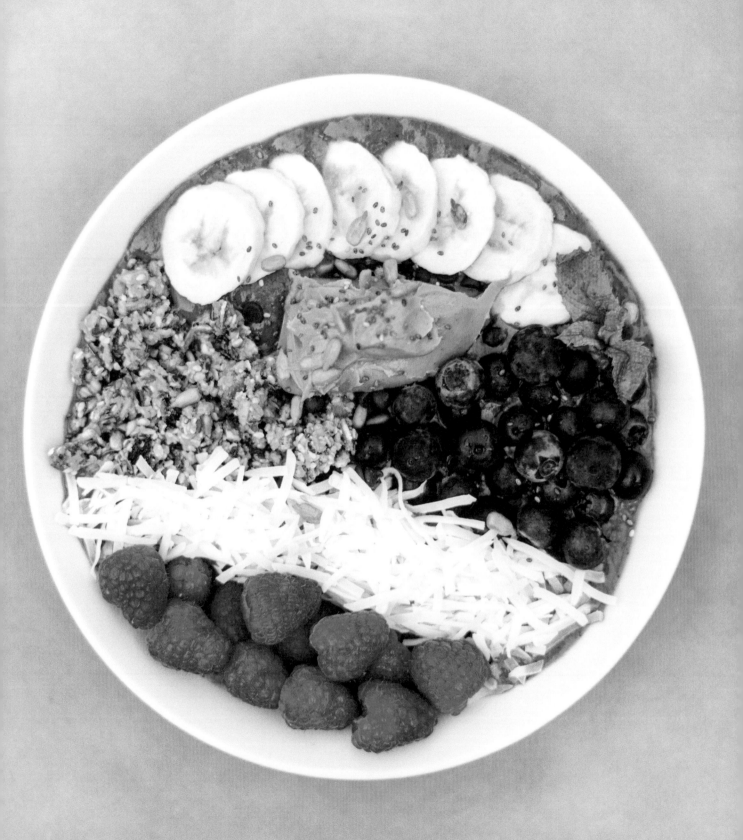

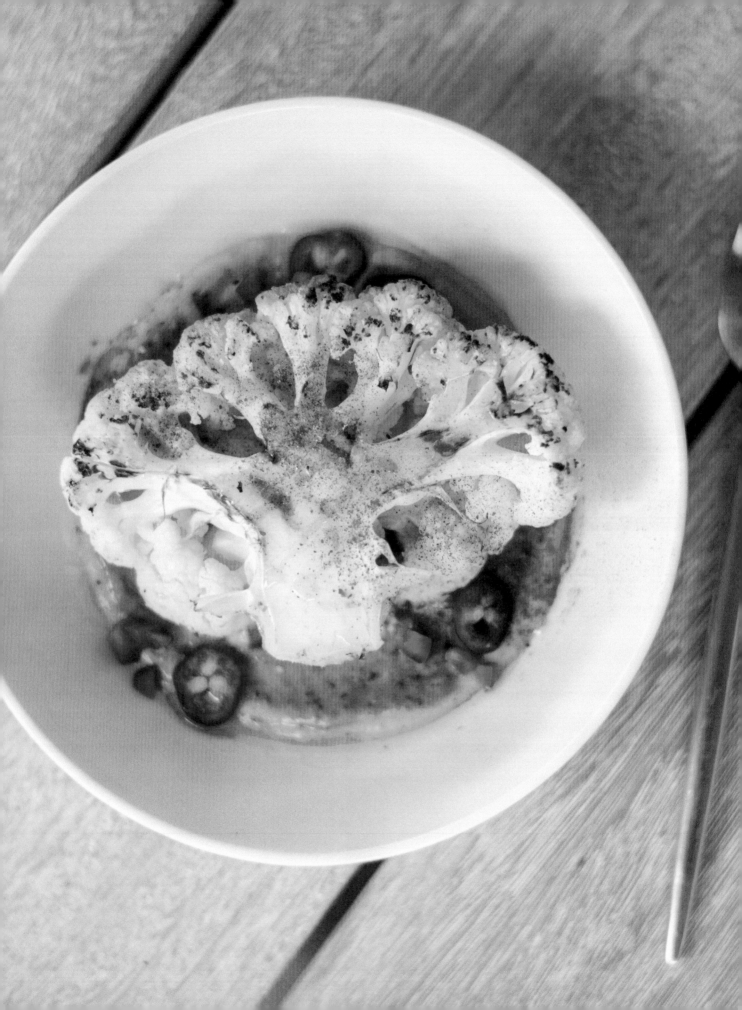

GRILLED CAULIFLOWER
WITH AVOCADO SALSA VERDE

Quite possibly, one of my fave ways to devour cauliflower.

Ingredients

1 head cauliflower

Olive oil

Chili lime seasoning

1 jar salsa verde

Avocado

Cilantro

Jalapeño (optional)

Directions

1. Preheat grill to medium heat, about 350°F.

2. Remove the outer leaves from the head of cauliflower. Then, using a large, sharp knife, cut the cauliflower in half. Brush each side with olive oil and season with chili lime.

3. Grill cauliflower on a covered grill for 5-6 minutes per side until cauliflower is tender and golden brown. Grilling time will vary based on the thickness of the cauliflower.

4. To a blender, add a jar of salsa verde, a diced avocado, and 1/3 cup of cilantro. Blend until smooth. For an extra kick, add a diced or grilled jalapeño before blending.

5. Plate cauliflower with a generous helping of avocado salsa verde and add this to your list of faves.

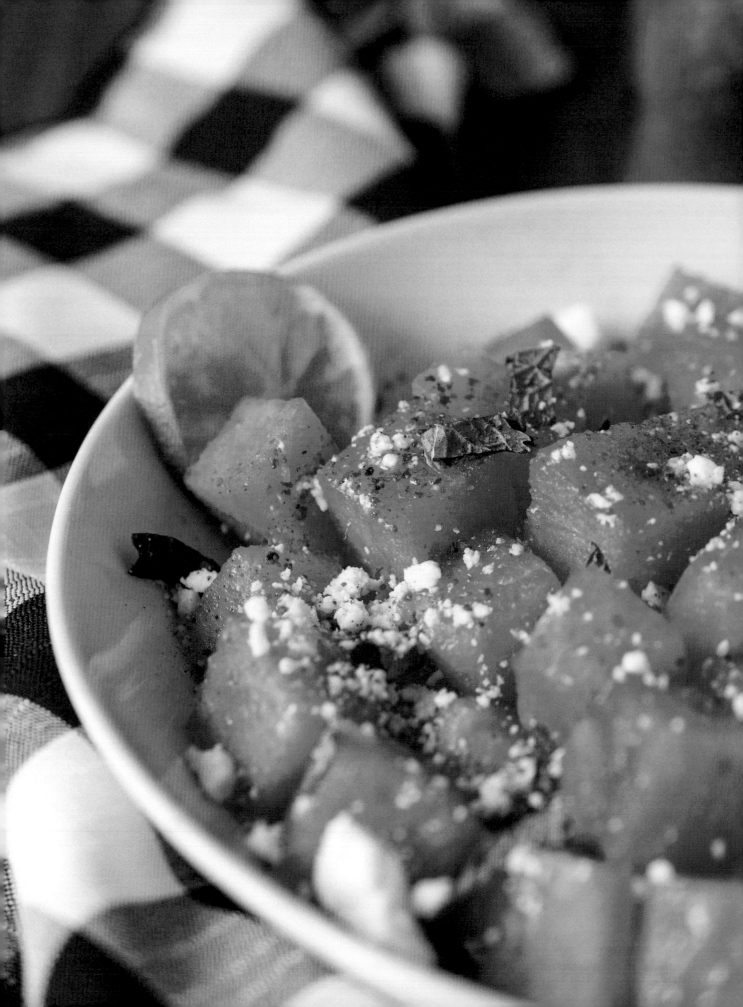

WATERMELON, MINT, AND FETA SALAD

She's just as tasty as she is pretty.

Ingredients

Watermelon

Fresh mint

Olive oil

Lime

Feta cheese

Chili lime seasoning

Directions

1. Cut watermelon into small cubes and place in a large bowl.

2. Chop mint and toss with watermelon.

3. Drizzle watermelon with olive oil and add a squeeze of lime juice.

4. Top salad with crumbled feta and a few dashes of chili lime.

5. Toss. Serve. #hostesswiththemostess

BACON AND PEANUT BUTTER

No, really, just bacon and peanut butter.

Ingredients

Bacon

Peanut butter

Directions

1. Preheat oven to 425°F and line a baking sheet with aluminum foil.

2. Arrange bacon on the baking sheet making sure the strips don't overlap.

3. Bake for 25 minutes or until it reaches the preferred level of crispiness.

4. Add a spoonful (or two) of peanut butter to a bowl and microwave for 1-2 minutes. Kick back, relax, and enjoy this tasty southern fare.

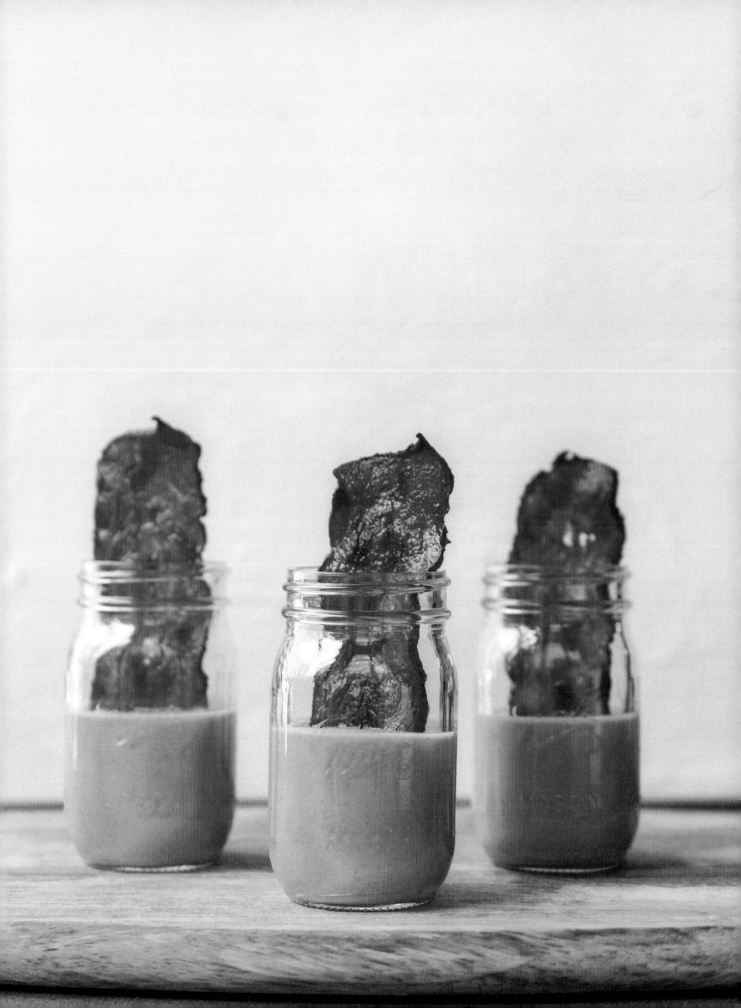

SEERSUCKER PROTEIN BALLS

Watch yourself with these bad boys. Next thing you know, you've eaten the entire batch.

Ingredients

1 ½ cups rolled oats

2 scoops vanilla protein powder

½ cup shredded coconut

1 cup chocolate chips

½ cup peanut butter or nut butter

1 tablespoon honey

¼ cup chia seeds

Cinnamon

Directions

1. Line a baking sheet with parchment paper.

2. Toss all of the ingredients into a large bowl with a couple of dashes of cinnamon. Then, get your hands nice and dirty and mix it all together.

3. Form the mixture into balls and place them on the baking sheet.

4. Chill protein balls in the fridge for 30 minutes.

Beth's Tip

Attention mamas: this is a great one to make with the kids!
Store leftovers in the fridge for healthy snacking all week long.

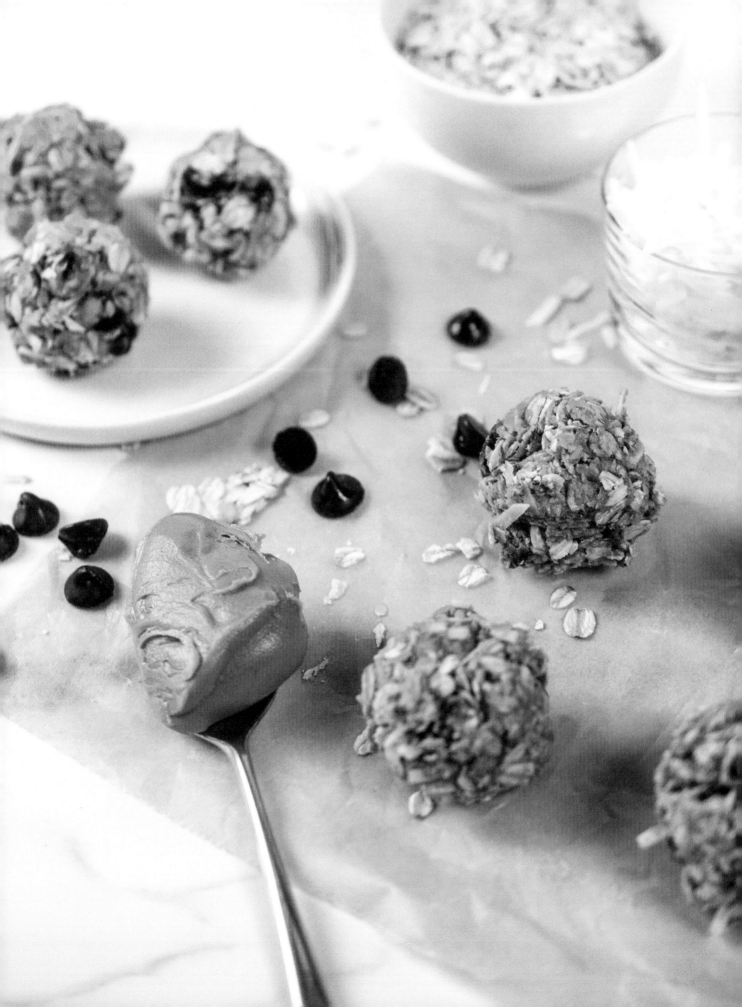

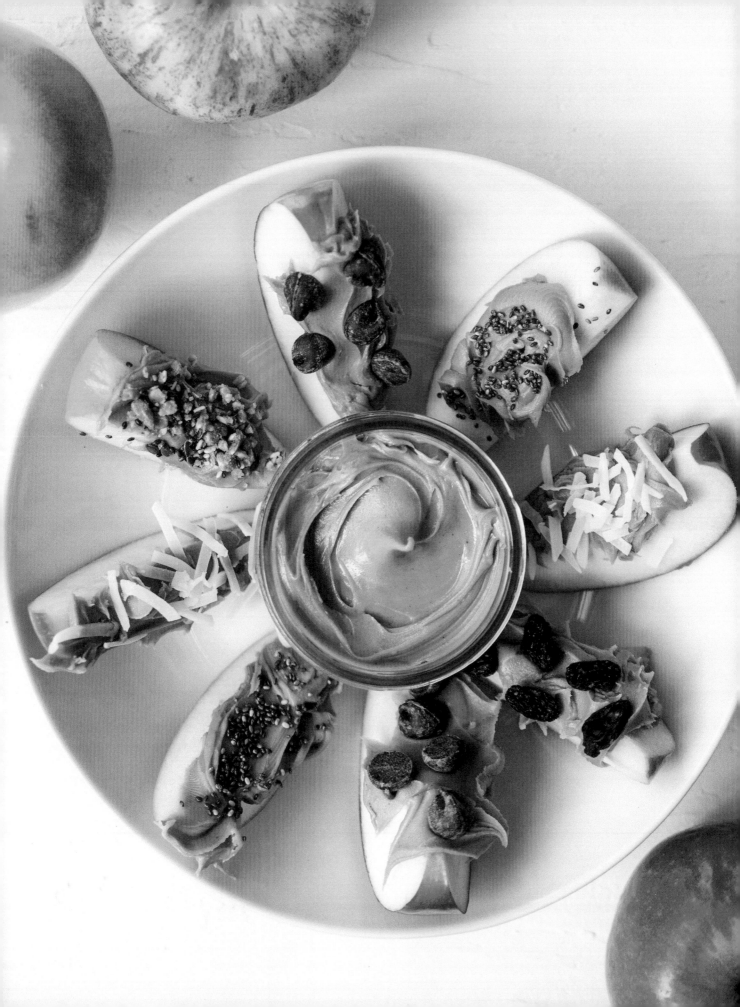

SNACK APPLES

Curb your sweet tooth with this easy-breezy snack.

Ingredients

Apples

Peanut butter or nut butter

Chia seeds

Unsweetened shredded coconut

Chocolate chips

Raisins

Dried cranberries

Trail mix

Directions

1. Cut apples into wedges.

2. Slather each apple slice with peanut butter.

3. Mix and mingle your toppings. No rules, just sweet snacking!

CHARCUTERIE BOARDS

The great thing about charcuterie boards is that they are easy to assemble, they're beautiful, and of course, they're delicious! Here are five tips from my friend and food stylist, Chung Chow, on how to up your charcuterie board game.

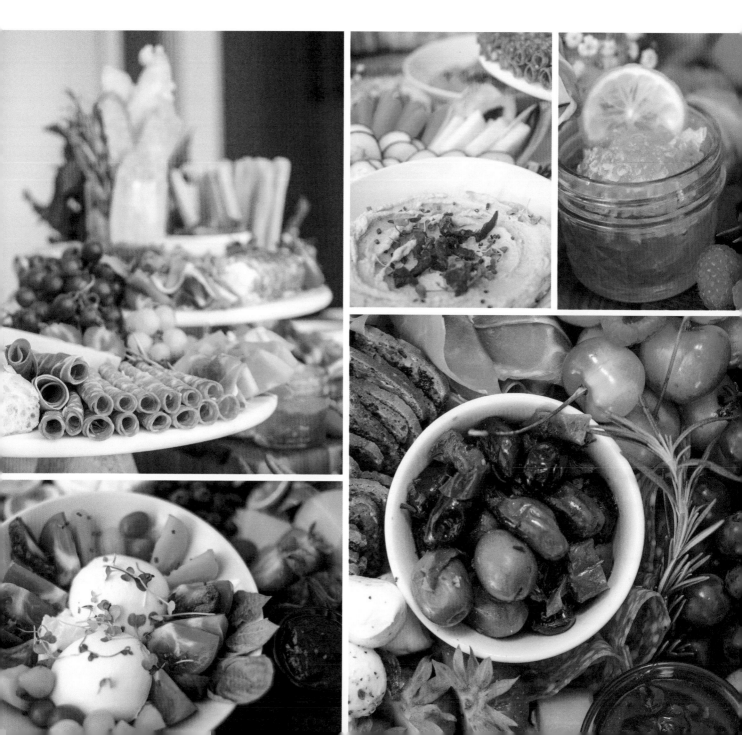

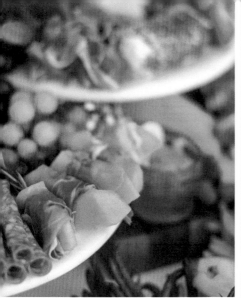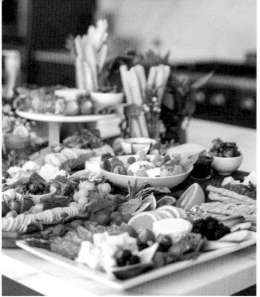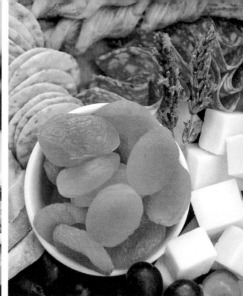

Variety – For charcuterie, select different styles of curing and cuts and take the time to display them in creative ways. Don't just remove meat from the package and plop it on the board. Roll thin cuts of soppressata into cigar shapes. Fold salami to give it a ribbon effect. Chop chorizo into cubes. Wrap prosciutto around sliced melon or crispy breadsticks. For cheese, have a variety of options ranging from hard, to semi-soft, to soft. The same rule applies here—slice it, crumble it, stack it. You get it.

Balance – Use something fresh or pickled to balance out the richness of the charcuterie and cheese. Grapes, pears, berries, nuts, cornichons, and olives all work well here. Use whatever you have in your pantry or what's in season.

Use those Bowls - Instead of putting jam, mustard, or honey directly on the board, use small bowls or ramekins. This small step makes a big difference when it comes to presentation.

Unexpected Extras – Add hummus with a variety of fresh veggies or a bowl of burrata with heirloom tomatoes, basil, and olive oil. Let your creativity shine with something tasty and non-traditional.

Finishing Touches – Elevate your charcuterie board with finishing salt, a drizzle of nice olive oil, fresh herbs, or edible flowers if you're feeling extra special.

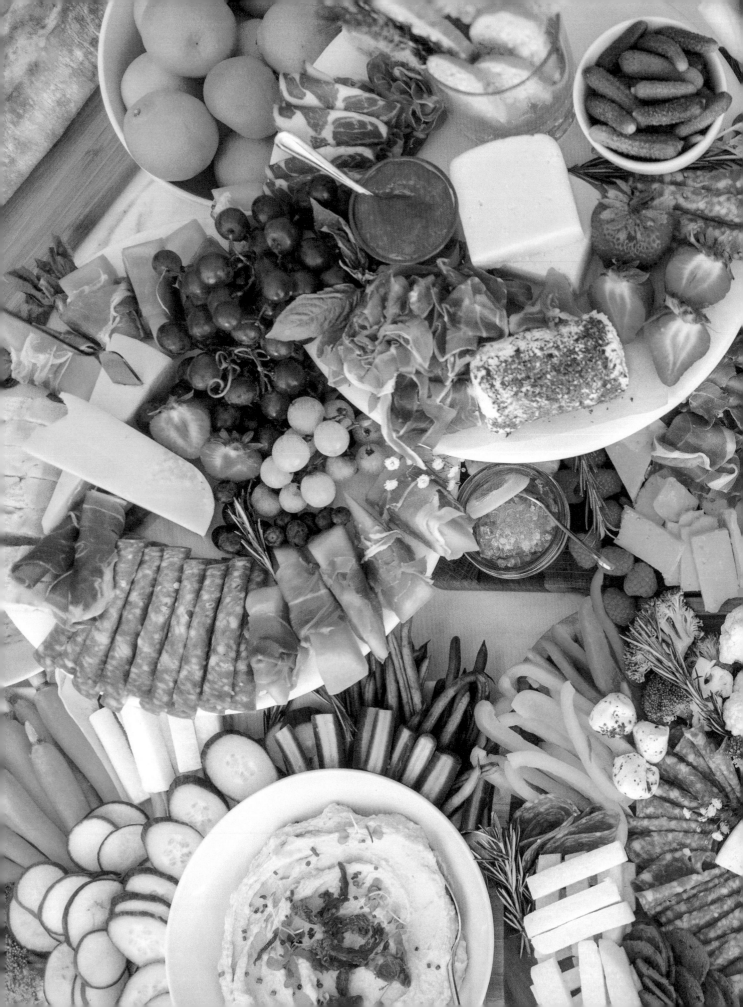

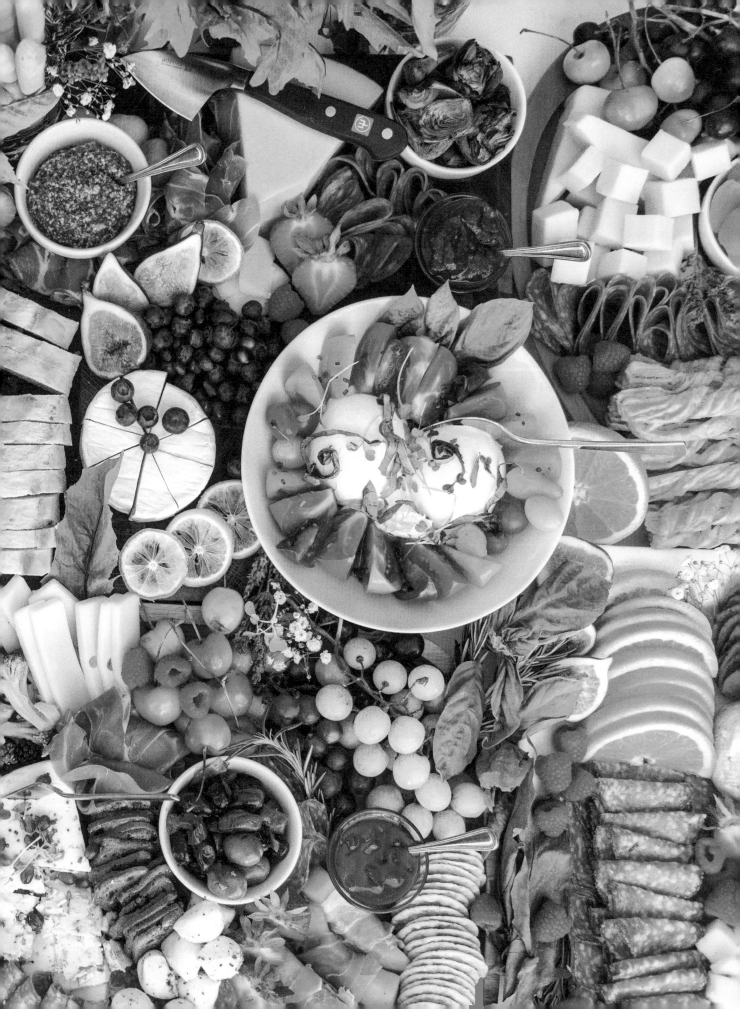

Chapter Four

THINK DRINK(S)

Smoothies, cocktails, juice!
I've got you covered for the weekdays...and the weekends.

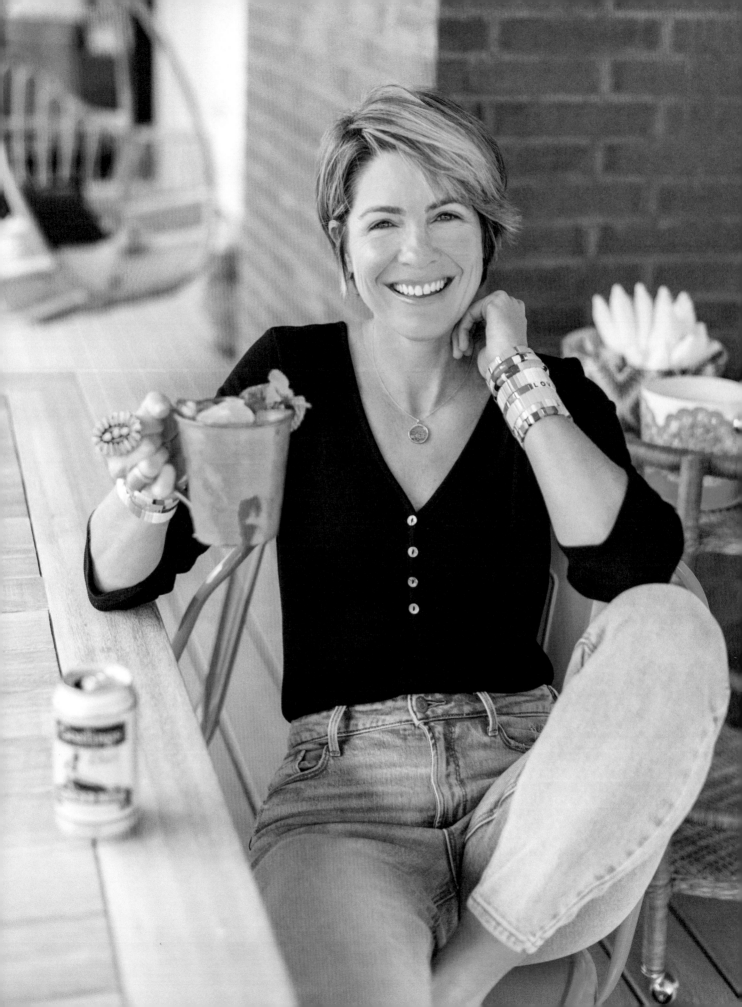

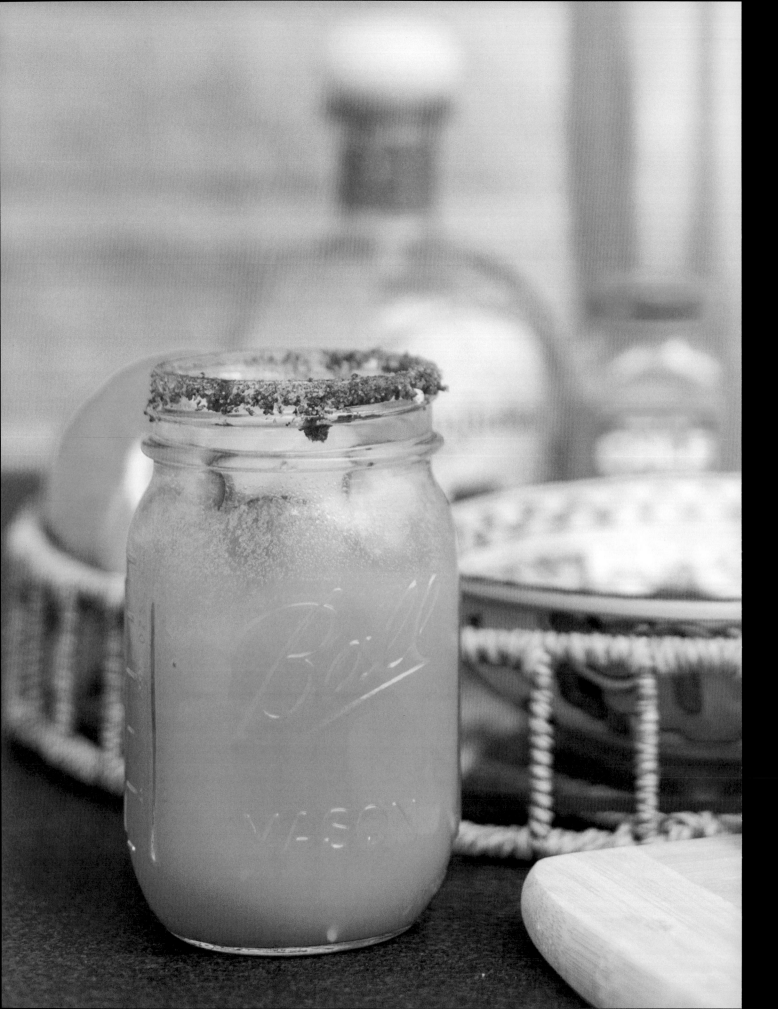

SPICY PALOMA

You had me at chili lime rim.

Ingredients

Grapefruit

Chili lime seasoning

Jalapeño

Tequila

Grapefruit sparkling water

Directions

1. Moisten the rim of glasses with grapefruit juice, then dip glasses in chili lime to make a spicy rim. Set aside.

2. In a cocktail shaker, muddle a jalapeño, add tequila, and the juice of one grapefruit and give it a good shake!

3. Serve over ice in a chili lime rimmed glass.

4. Top with sparkling water and toast to the good life!

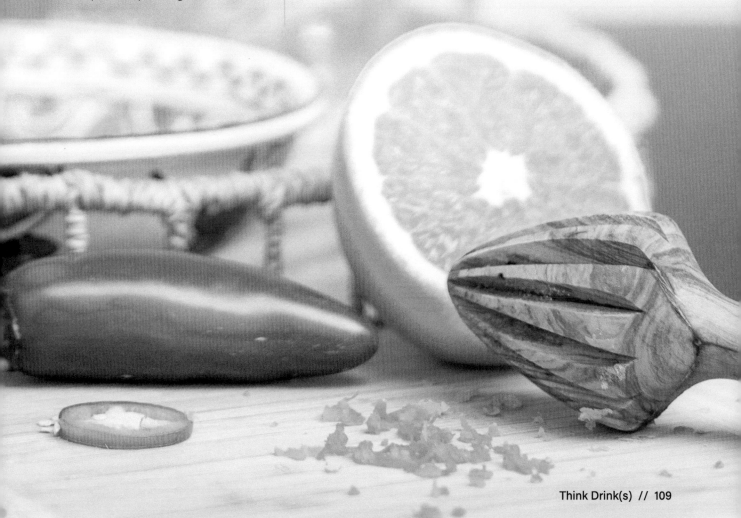

LOW-CARB MOSCOW MULE

Enjoy this baby with zero guilt.

Ingredients

½ ounce lime juice

1 ½ ounces vodka

4 ounces diet ginger beer

Ice

Lime, for garnish

Mint, for garnish

Directions

1. Pour lime juice, vodka, and ginger beer into a moscow mule mug and stir gently.

2. Add ice and garnish with mint and lime. Cheers it up and enjoy!

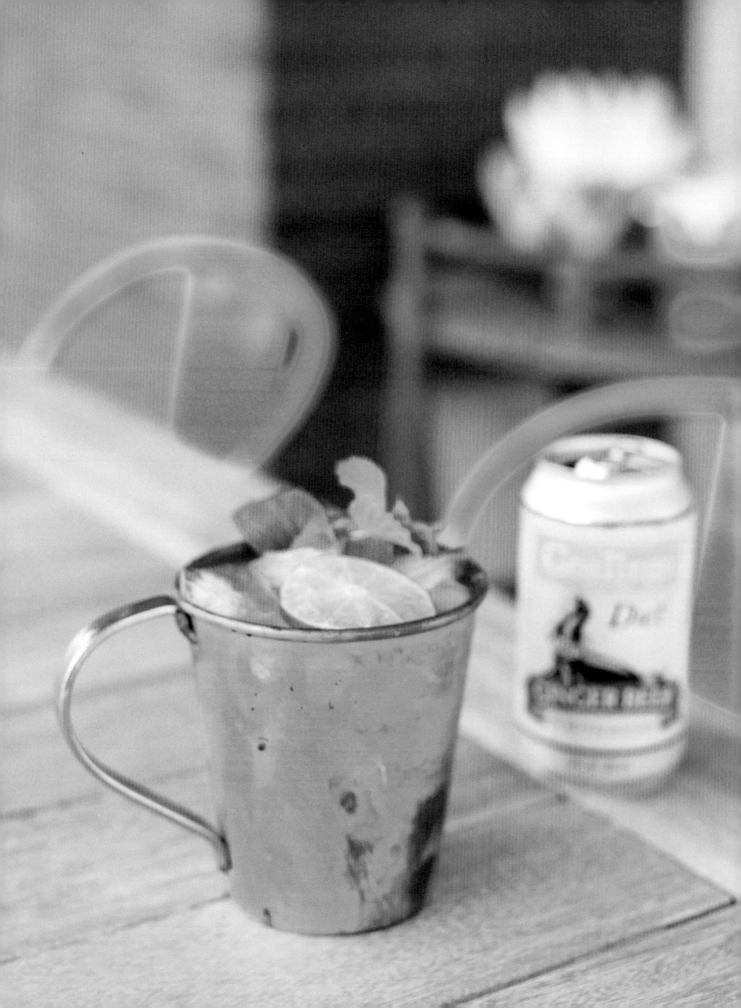

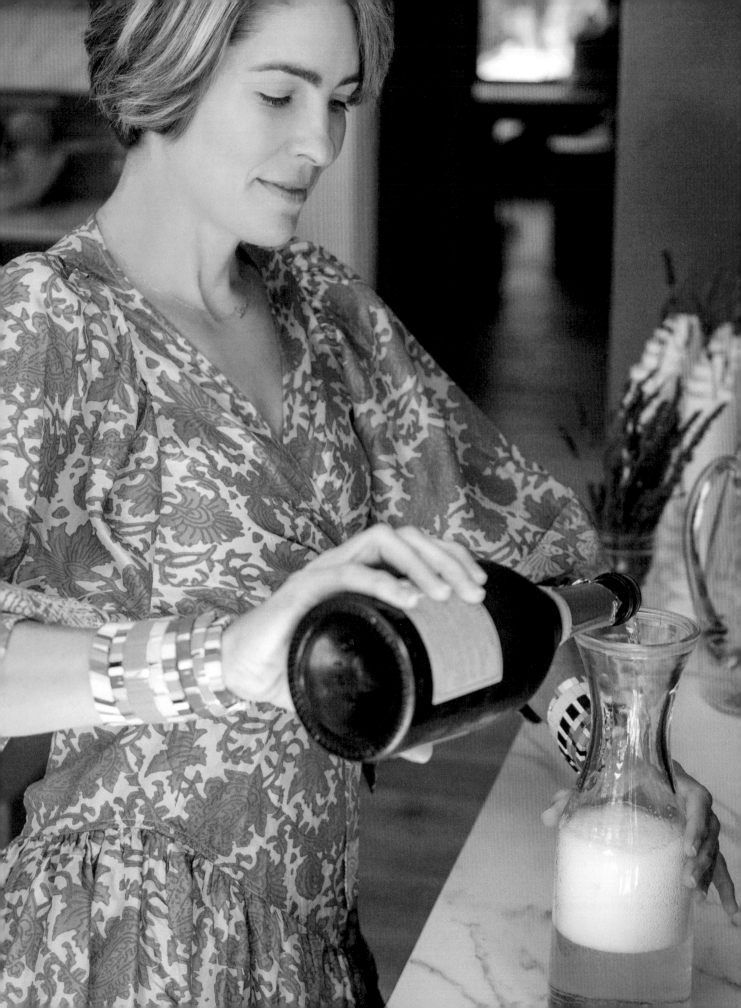

LAVENDER PROSECCO

This is a libation you bust out for your special occasions.

Ingredients

1 cup water

1 cup sugar

Lavender sprigs

Prosecco

Directions

1. Combine water, sugar, and lavender in a small saucepan. Bring to a boil and stir until sugar dissolves.

2. Remove from heat and let lavender syrup steep for 30 minutes. Remove lavender sprigs and let the syrup cool. Chill until ready to use.

3. When it's time to serve, fill champagne glasses 3/4 full with chilled prosecco. Top with lavender simple syrup.

4. Add a sprig of lavender to garnish and watch your party-goers enjoy this beautiful bubbly cocktail.

Beth's Tip

I snagged my lavender at my local nursery.

GREEN JUICE

Imagine sipping this overlooking the Italian coast. That's where I first discovered this deliciousness.

Ingredients

½ bunch celery

Whole pineapple

2 granny smith apples

1-inch piece fresh ginger

Directions

1. Wash and quarter the celery.

2. Chop the pineapple into large pieces.

3. Wash and quarter the apples.

4. Push celery, pineapple, apples, and ginger through the juicer.

5. Drink immediately! LA BELLA VITA.

Beth's Tip

Traveling to the Amalfi Coast? Definitely hit up Casa Angelina.

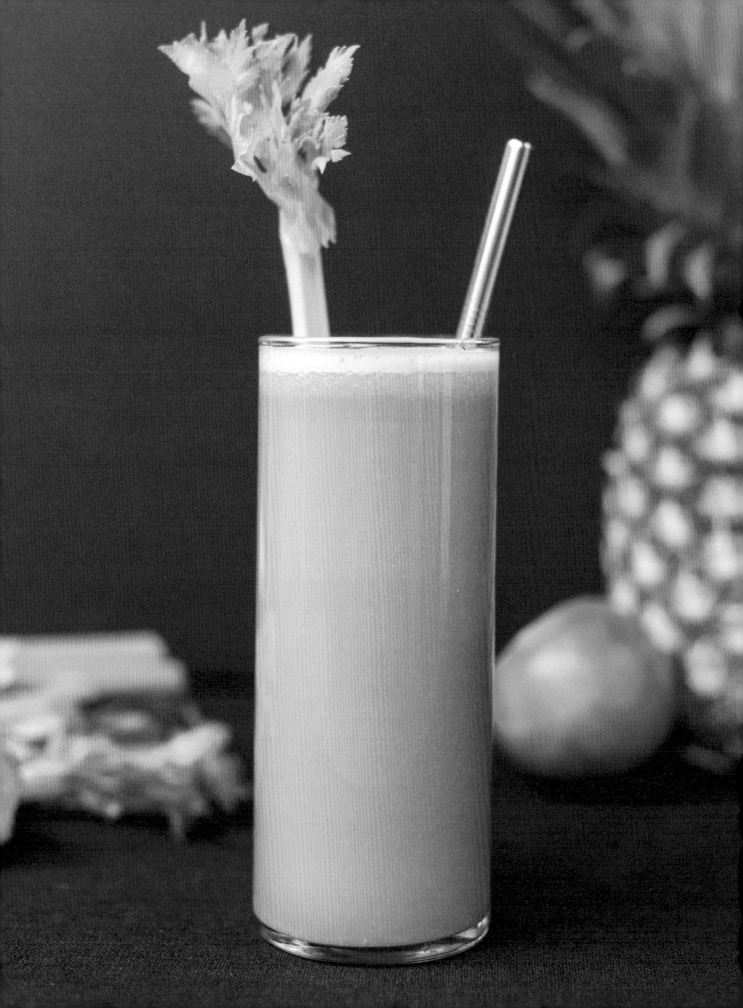

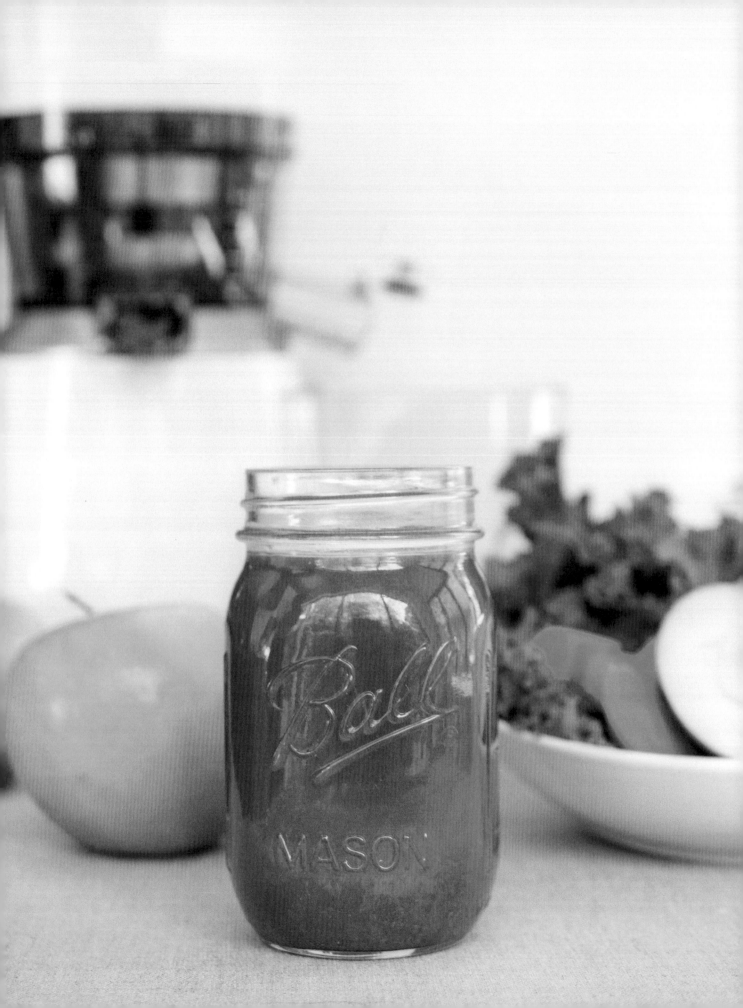

BETTER THAN IT LOOKS JUICE

Don't judge a juice by its color.

Ingredients

3 carrots

3 celery stalks

Handful of kale

2 granny smith apples

Cinnamon

1-inch piece fresh ginger

Directions

1. Wash and quarter carrots and celery.

2. Chop kale into large pieces.

3. Wash and quarter apples. Sprinkle with cinnamon.

4. Push veggies, apples, and ginger through the juicer.

Beth's Tip

I love drinking this juice on a regular macro day.
It's chock full of healthy carbs.

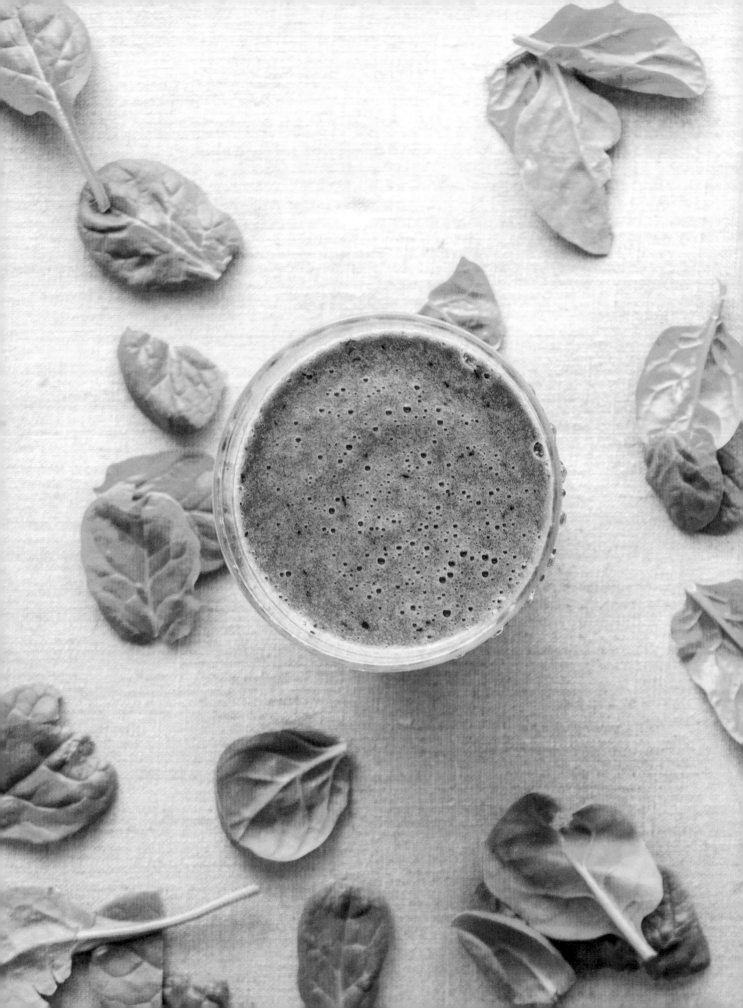

GREEN MONSTER

Good on regular macro days and a hit with the kids too.

Ingredients

Baby spinach

Banana, frozen

Blueberries

Vanilla protein powder

Coconut water

Directions

Add a handful of baby spinach, one chopped frozen banana, a handful of blueberries, a scoop of protein powder, and coconut water to a blender. Blend until smooth. Sip in all those nutrients!

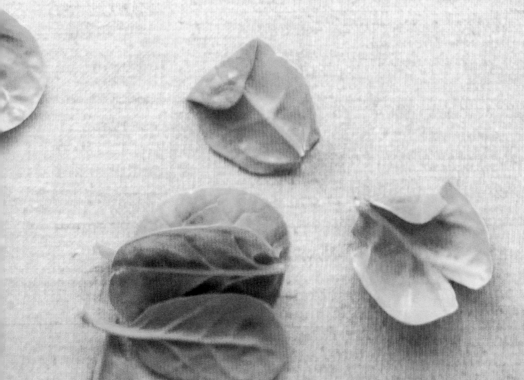

DATE PEANUT BUTTER SMOOTHIE

This milkshake brings all the kids to the yard!

Ingredients

4-5 pitted dates

1 cup unsweetened almond milk

1 banana, frozen

1 spoonful peanut butter

Vanilla protein powder

Ice

Directions

Soak dates in hot water for 5-10 minutes. Drain. Add all of the ingredients to a blender with a handful of crushed ice. Blend until smooth. This legit rivals a caramel milkshake.

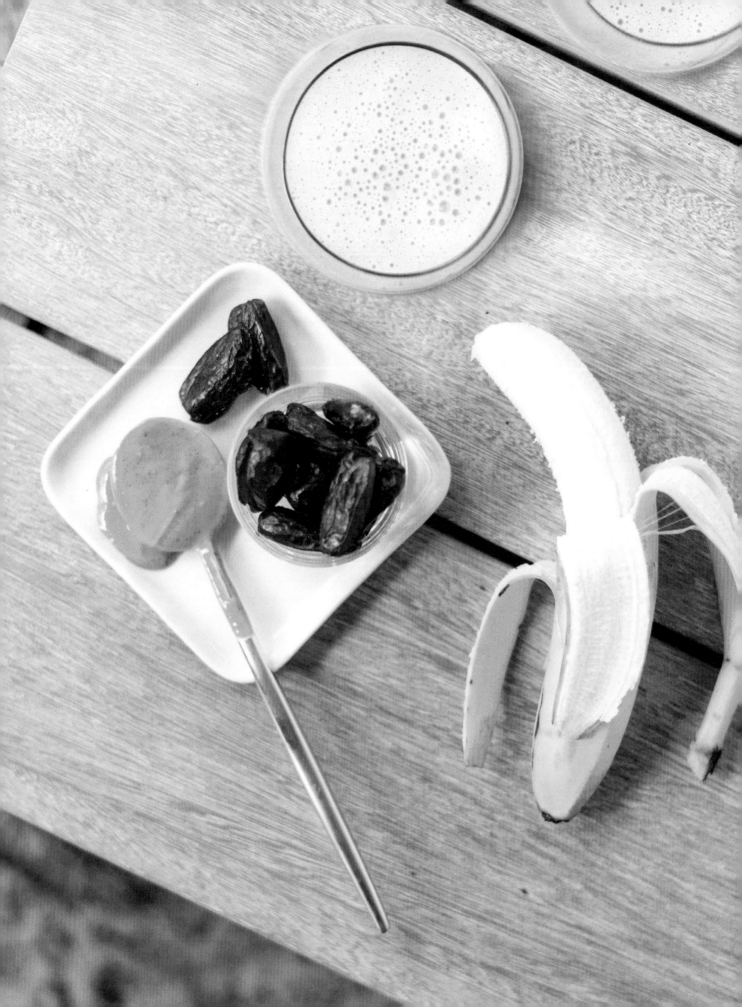

CHAI BANANA PROTEIN DRINK

Chai tea latte lovers rejoice!

Ingredients

Chai latte concentrate

Banana, frozen

Vanilla protein powder

Cinnamon

Ice

Directions

Pour chai latte concentrate into a blender. Add remaining ingredients to a blender with a handful of crushed ice. Blend until smooth. And skip that afternoon drive-thru!

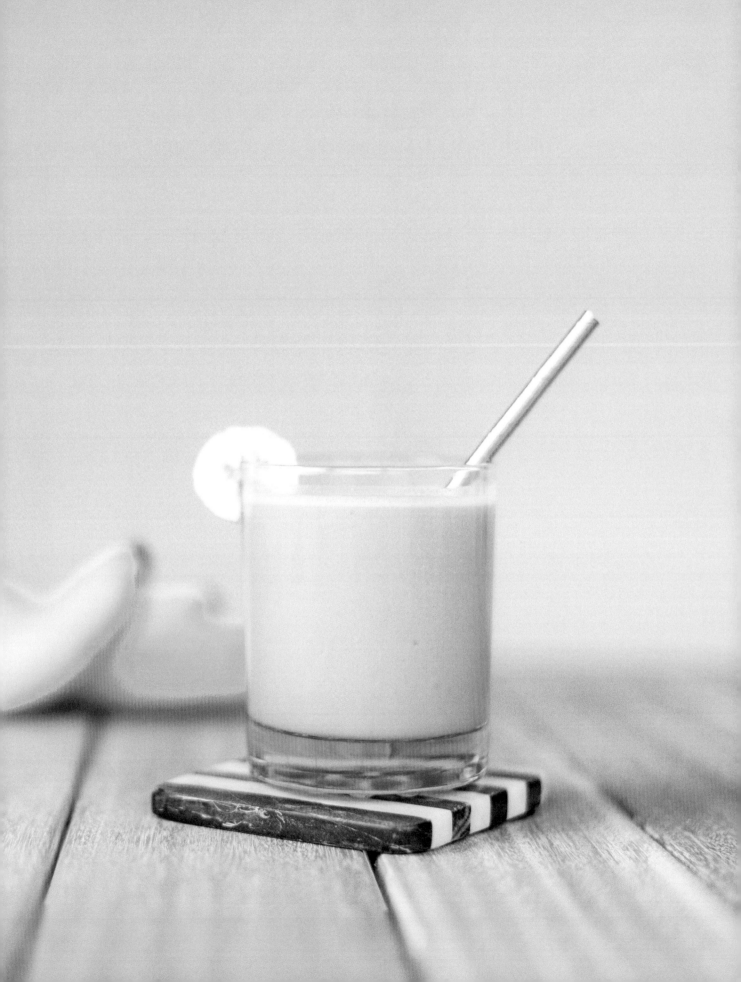

CHOCOLATE PEANUT BUTTER PROTEIN SHAKE

That time a PB cup married a protein shake.

Ingredients

Chocolate protein powder

Coconut water

1 spoonful peanut butter

Ice

Directions

Add all ingredients to blender with a handful of crushed ice and blend until smooth.

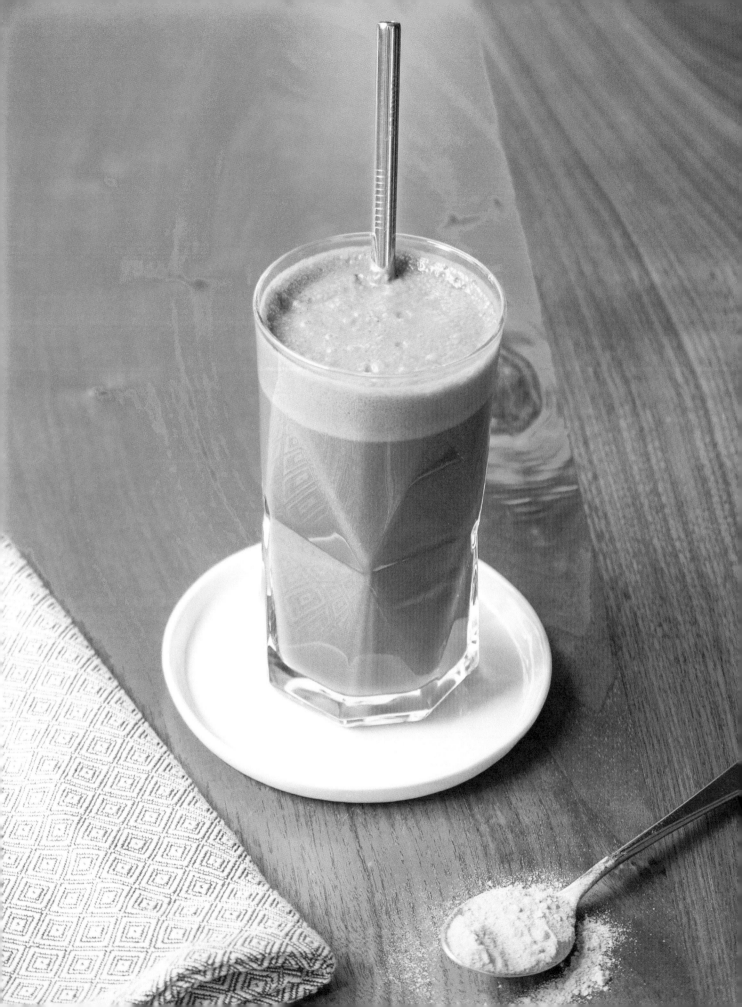

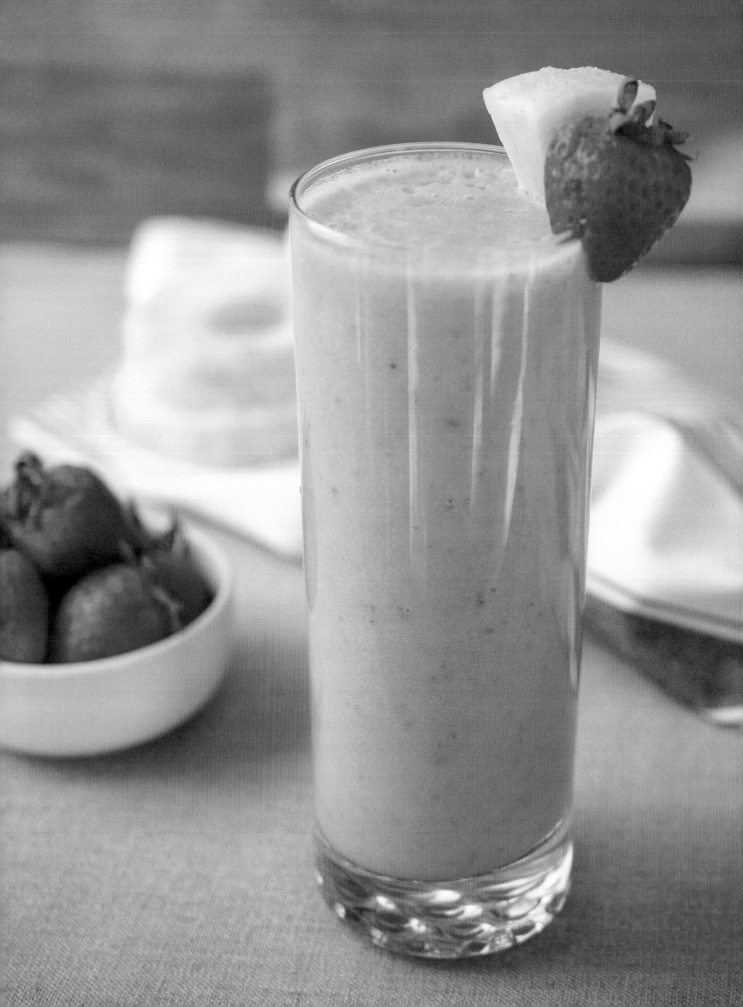

TROPICAL PROTEIN SMOOTHIE

Don't forget your pineapple. It's the star of the show.

Ingredients

4 strawberries

1 banana

Pineapple chunks

Vanilla protein powder

Coconut water

Ice

Directions

Add strawberries, chopped banana, a handful of pineapple chunks, a scoop of protein powder, coconut water, and a handful of crushed ice to a blender. Blend until smooth.

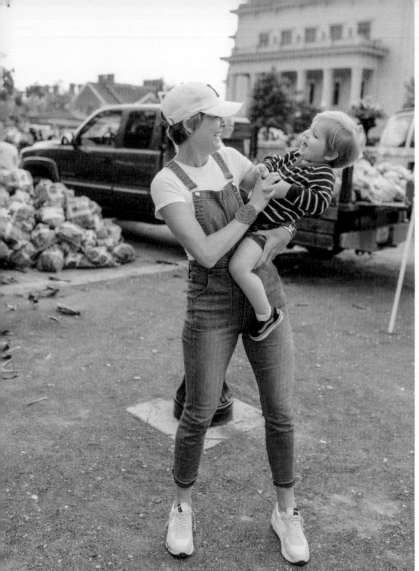
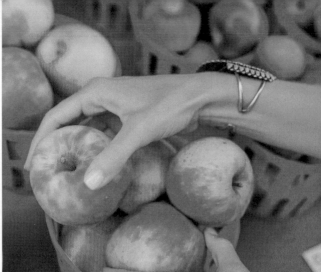
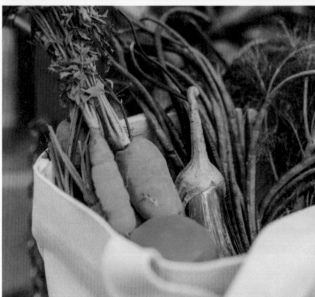

THE FARMERS MARKET

One of my favorite spring and summer traditions is the Saturday morning farmers market. Lucky for us Midwesterners, we have some gems. I am typically up with Calvin before the rest of the house, so I love this time with just the two of us. Sometimes I let him roam free. Other times we stroll. But we always stock up on some stellar locally grown produce and DONUTS. Think kale, tomatoes, corn, eggplant, herbs, olive oils, squash, strawberries, peaches, and honey, to name a few.

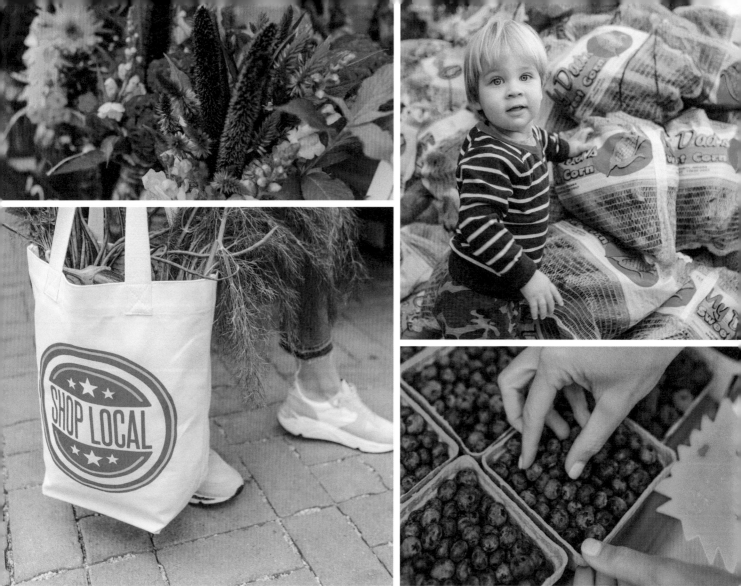

On the off chance the girls are up, they tag along, which I find motivates them to eat the healthy goodies they pick out! I love meeting the farmers, hearing their stories, and supporting their businesses. But most importantly, I love serving up their delicious goodies to my family—in a bowl.

Chapter Five

#MOMHACKS

Let's face it...life is busy. Let Mama help you out.

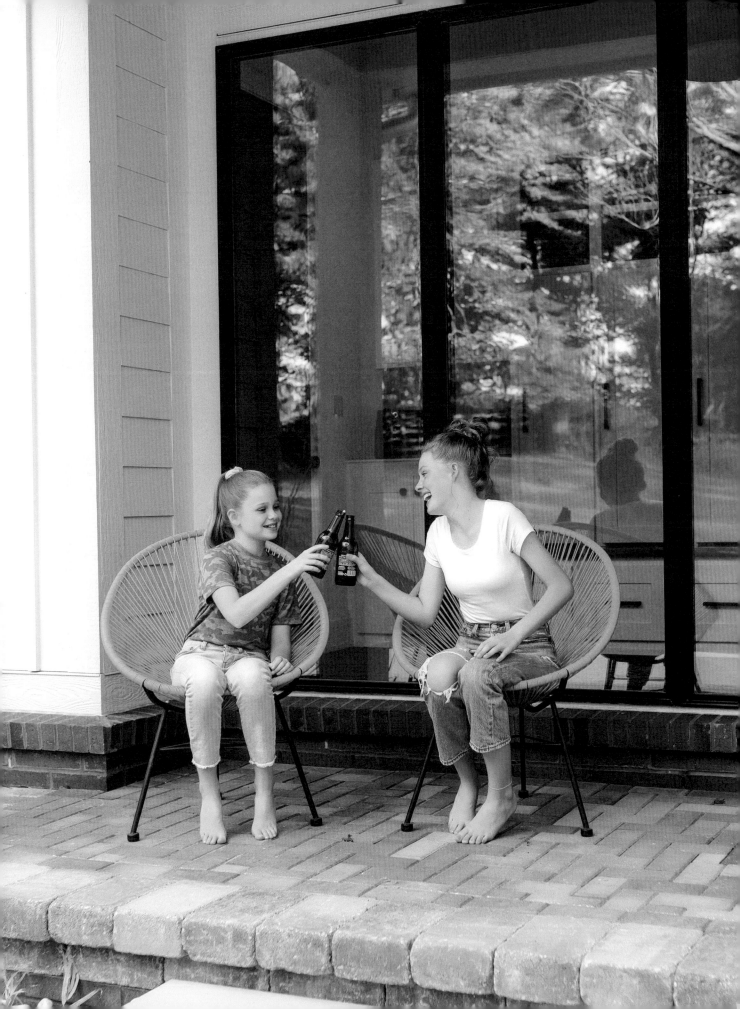

Beth's Tip

If you feel like you need butter for your potato,
try a little coconut oil.

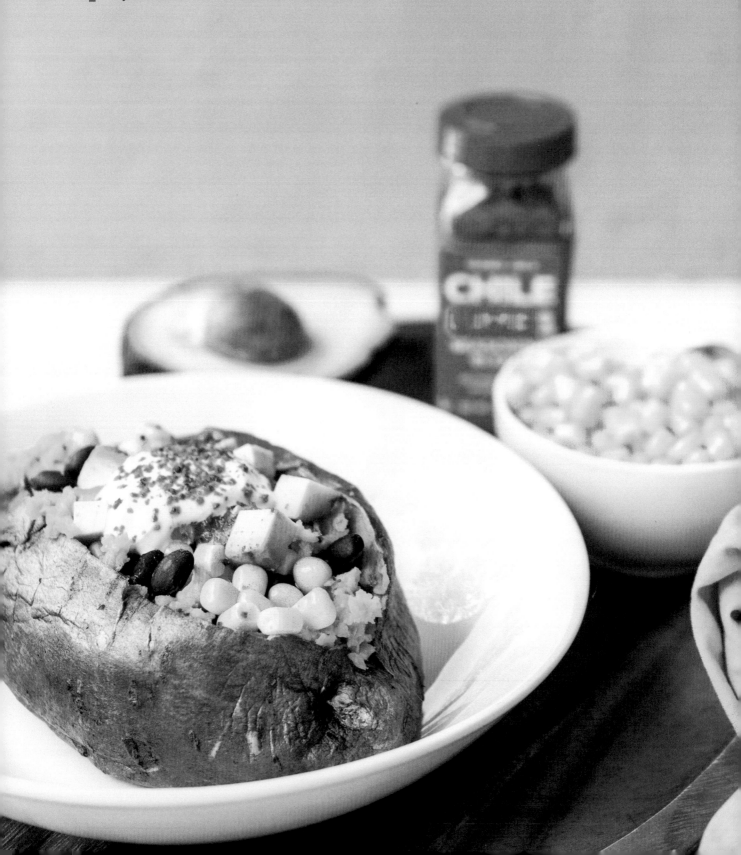

MEXI-TATER

You can bake these taters if you have an hour, but if you're against the clock,
you can also microwave everything, and it's just as delish.

Ingredients

Sweet potato

Coconut oil

Corn

Black beans

Avocado

Chili lime seasoning

Jalapeños

Greek yogurt

Directions

1. Wash tater and rub with coconut oil. Stab all over with a fork and microwave for 10 minutes.

2. Drain corn and beans, season with chili lime, and heat in the microwave

3. Chop avocado and season with chili lime.

4. Chop jalapeños.

5. Slice tater down the middle. Top with beans, corn, avocado, a dollop of greek yogurt, jalapeños, and an extra dash of chili lime. Carb-loaded, flavor-filled, and EASY.

SNEAKY VEGGIE SAUCE

Picky eaters? This sauce will win them over.

Ingredients

Marinara sauce

Baby spinach

Olive oil

1-2 cloves of garlic, minced

Salt and pepper

Italian seasoning

Pasta, for serving—preferably gluten free

Directions

1. Add marinara sauce and a big ol' handful of baby spinach to a bullet or blender and blend until smooth.

2. Heat olive oil in a saucepan over medium-high heat. Add minced garlic, and do a quick sauté. Add blended marinara sauce. Season to taste with salt, pepper, and italian seasoning.

3. Bring sauce to a boil and then lower the heat to keep the sauce at a simmer. Simmer for 10-15 minutes.

4. Serve over pasta and remember, what they don't know can't hurt 'em.

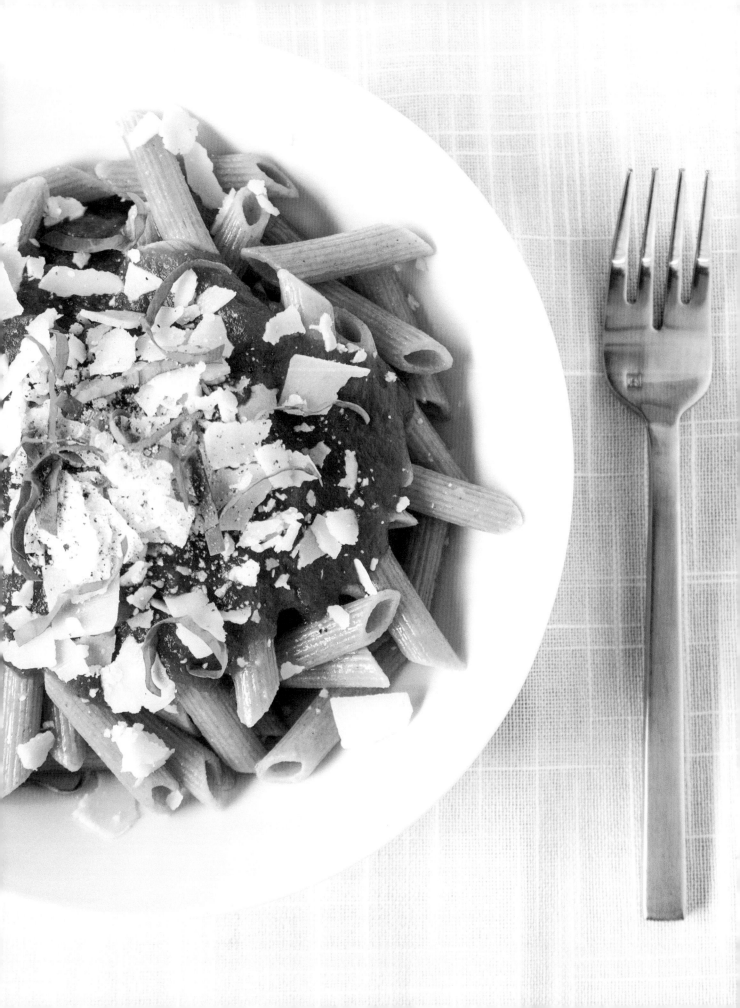

CHICKEN VEGETABLE SOUP HACK

Delicious, easy, soup in 5 minutes? Yes, please!

Ingredients

Premade veggie soup, your favorite type

Rotisserie chicken

Toppings:

Avocado

Greek yogurt

Shredded cheese

Jalapeños

Directions

Heat soup and add chopped rotisserie chicken. Add your fave toppings and enjoy this hearty goodness. #nobrainer

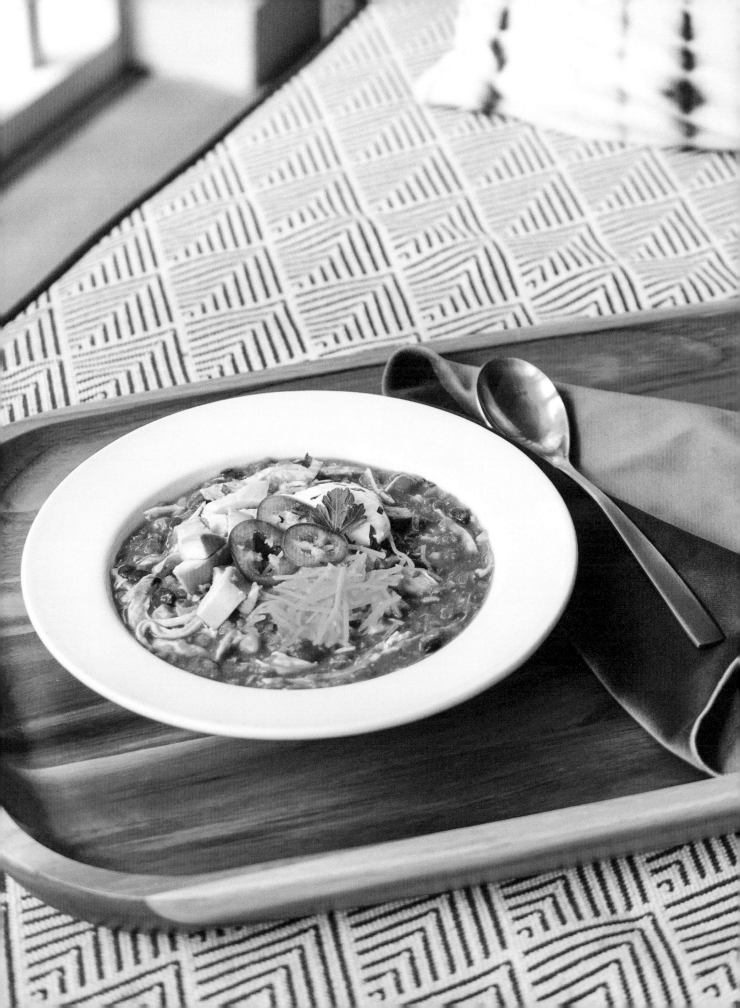

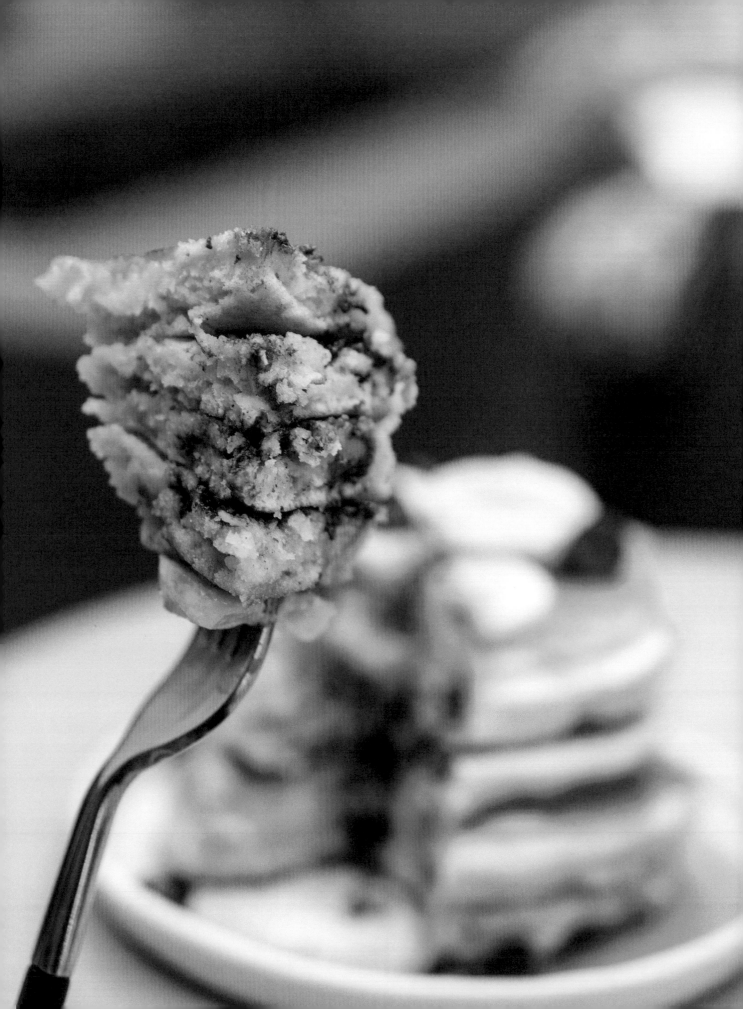

BANANA DATE CINNAMON PANCAKES

Is it dessert or breakfast? Your kids will never know!

Ingredients

5 dates

Pancake mix

1 banana

Cinnamon

Vanilla protein powder

Coconut oil

Maple syrup

Directions

1. Soak dates in hot water for 5 minutes. Drain.

2. To a blender, add pancake mix and liquid, according to the package directions for one batch of batter.

3. Add dates, chopped banana, a dash of cinnamon, and a scoop of vanilla protein powder. Blend until smooth.

4. Heat coconut oil in a large skillet or on a griddle over medium-high heat. Drop batter onto griddle and cook until the outside is crisp and the middle is fluffy. Flipping halfway through.

5. Drizzle with maple syrup and watch the kids devour these cakes!

Beth's Tip

Feeling frisky, add chocolate chips to your pancakes after you drop batter onto the griddle.

CHIA ON THE GO

The easiest and cutest on-the-go snack!

Ingredients

Almond Milk

Chia Seeds

Honey

Bananas

Pineapple

Strawberries

Blueberries

Granola

Shredded coconut

Dried mango slices (optional)

Directions

The Night Before

1. In a large bowl, stir together 2 cups almond milk, 1 cup chia seeds, and a squeeze of honey.

2. Put the mixture in a mason jar, cover with plastic wrap, and place in the fridge overnight.

3. In the morning, give the mixture a good stir. It will have thickened to a pudding consistency.

At the Table

Toss pudding into a bowl. Layer chopped fresh fruit, granola, and shredded coconut on top of the pudding. Spruce it up with some dried fruit if you prefer.

Headed Out

Keep pudding in the jar. Layer chopped fresh fruit, granola and shredded coconut on top of the pudding. Ready, set, goodness on-the-go!

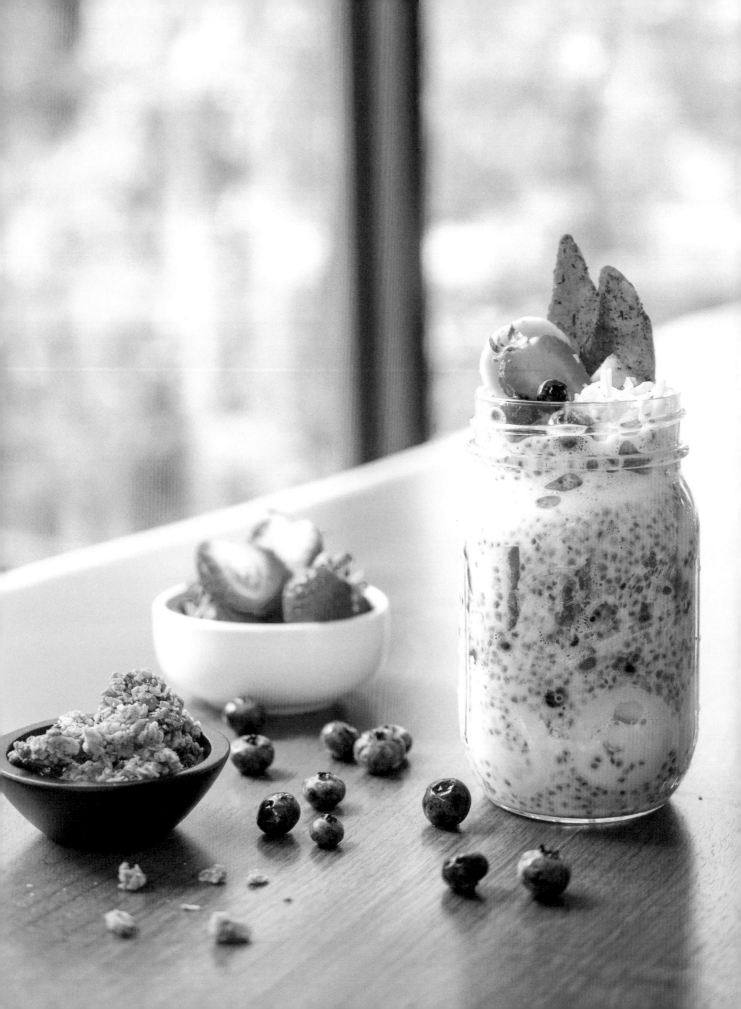

NO-BAKE PEANUT BUTTERSCOTCH
PROTEIN COOKIES

One of Nonnie's sweet treats that's ready in no time!

Ingredients

1 bag butterscotch chips

1 cup peanut butter

2 cups peanuts

Vanilla protein powder

Directions

1. In a microwave-safe bowl, melt butterscotch chips.

2. Add peanut butter and stir to combine.

3. Add peanuts and a scoop of protein powder and give it another good stir.

4. Drop large dollops onto a baking sheet lined with wax paper.

5. Place in freezer for 15-20 minutes. You've been forewarned, these are addictive!

Beth's Tip

Double this recipe—I do!

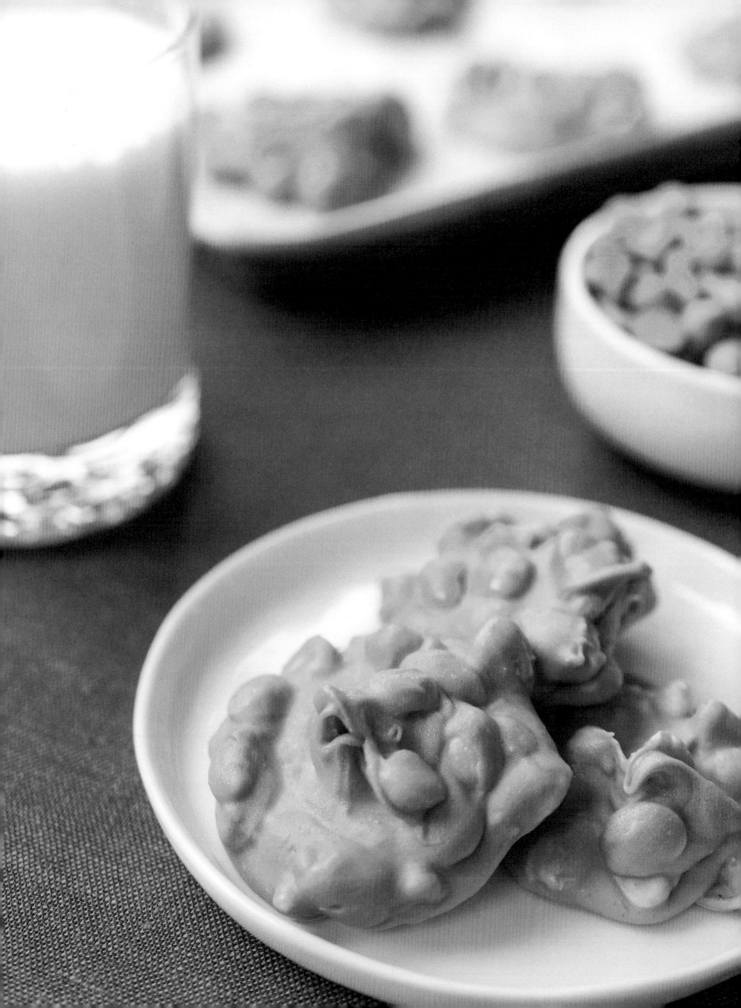

SAMMY MELTS

When I truly don't feel like cooking, this is a crowd-pleasing meal for the entire fam.

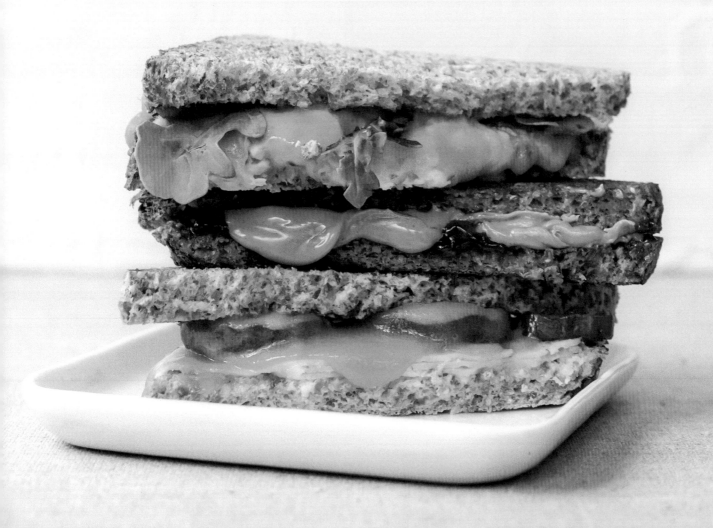

TUNA MELT

Ingredients

Canned Tuna

Mayo

Red Onion

Everything bagel seasoning

Whole grain hearty bread

Sliced Cheese

Arugula

Directions

1. Make tuna salad: drain tuna and break it up with your hands. Add 2-3 spoonfuls of mayo, diced red onion, and bagel seasoning.

2. Pop two slices of bread into the toaster. When toasted, spread each slice with mayo.

3. Add tuna salad to one slice of bread, slap on a piece of cheese and stick it under the broiler for a hot minute until the cheese melts.

4. Top with a little arugula and the second slice of bread.

PB&J MELT

Whole grain hearty bread

Coconut Oil

Cinnamon

Peanut butter

Fruit preserves

1. Spread coconut oil on the outside of each slice of bread, sprinkle with cinnamon.

2. Then, just like mom did, make your PB and J.

3. Heat large skillet or griddle over medium-high heat and cook your sammy until golden brown on both sides.

TURKEY MELT

Whole grain hearty bread

Dijon mustard

Mayo

Deli Turkey

Pickles

Sliced cheese

1. Pop two slices of bread into the toaster. When toasted, add dijon and mayo to one slice.

2. Layer with turkey, pickles, and cheese.

3. Pop under the broiler until the cheese melts. Be sure to watch it!

4. Top with the second slice of bread.

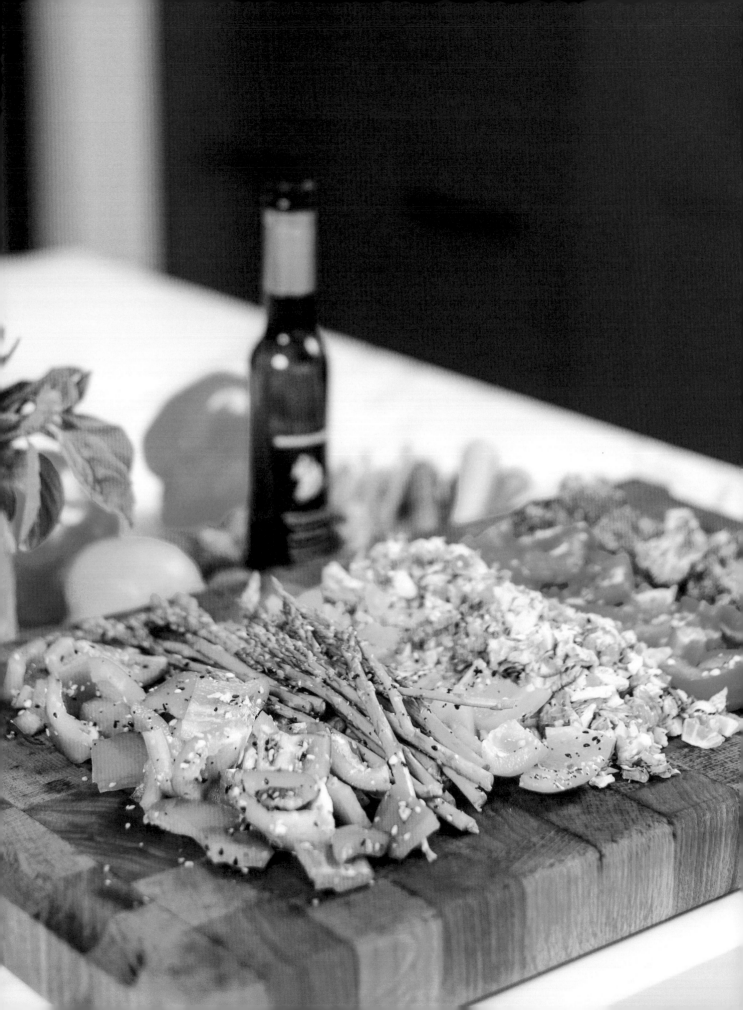

MEAL PREP

I'm about a 50/50 meal prepper. I have to say, it does indeed help in keeping me on track with my eats. It takes the guesswork out, you know?! So here's how and what I typically prep:

Chicken

Cook it up *"Seersucker Style"* (pg 16). Reheat chicken in the oven or in a skillet with olive oil.

Cauliflower Rice

This is my favorite bowl base! Roast it at 425°F for 25 minutes. Do a quick reheat in the oven, skillet, or microwave.

Fruit

Rinse your fruit, so it's ready for your sweet tooth cravings. Toss some in the freezer for protein smoothies! Peel your bananas before you freeze.

Pasta

Grab your gluten free pasta and cook according to directions.

Grains

I use the 90-sec microwaveable packs of quinoa or brown rice so, no prep needed. If you don't, cook up a big batch of grains. Reheat in a skillet, but the microwave won't kill it either!

Vegetables

Roast a variety of veggies at 425°F for 25 minutes. Reheat as you would your proteins. Chop fresh veggies for *Snacky Plates* (pg 85).

Hard-boiled Eggs

Make a large batch of eggs for snacking throughout the week.

Pasta Sauce

Sneaky Veggie Tomato Sauce (pg 134). Have this on hand for pasta, veggies, or chicken. It'll keep for the week!

Trail Mix

Mix all the nuts you like with shredded coconut, cacao nibs, and dried fruit. Another great on-the-go snack that you truly CAN'T MESS UP!

Tuna Salad

Make a big batch with bagel seasoning and mayo. Great stuffed in peppers, on wholegrain toast, or on crackers for a *Snacky Plate* (pg 85).

Chapter Six

THERE'S NO "I" IN
TEAM

Let's share the love!
These are some favorite recipes from the lovely
ladies that helped make #thatbowllife possible.

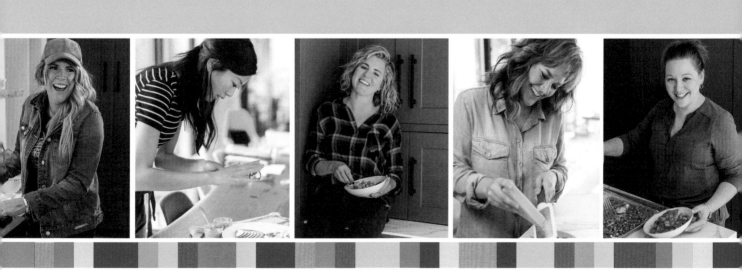

ASHLEY'S SALMON SALAD

Ashley Wittmer, Photography

I've had it. I loved it. And you will too.

Ingredients

2 cups cooked salmon, flaked

2 hard-boiled eggs, chopped

½ cucumber, diced

1 bell pepper, diced

2 green onions, diced

Capers (optional)

Salt and pepper

¼ teaspoon smoked paprika

Mayo

Cayenne pepper

Lemon

Everything bagel seasoning

Directions

1. In a large bowl, mix together flaked salmon, hard-boiled eggs, bell pepper, cucumber, green onions, and a spoonful of capers.

2. Season with salt, a generous grind of black pepper, and smoked paprika.

3. In a separate bowl, make the dressing by combining, 4-5 tablespoons of mayo, a dash of cayenne, and the juice of half a lemon.

4. Pour dressing over salmon and mix to combine.

5. Serve on a bed of arugula or with cucumber slices and other fresh veggies. Top with a dash of bagel seasoning.

Beth's Tip

This is a great way to use leftover salmon.

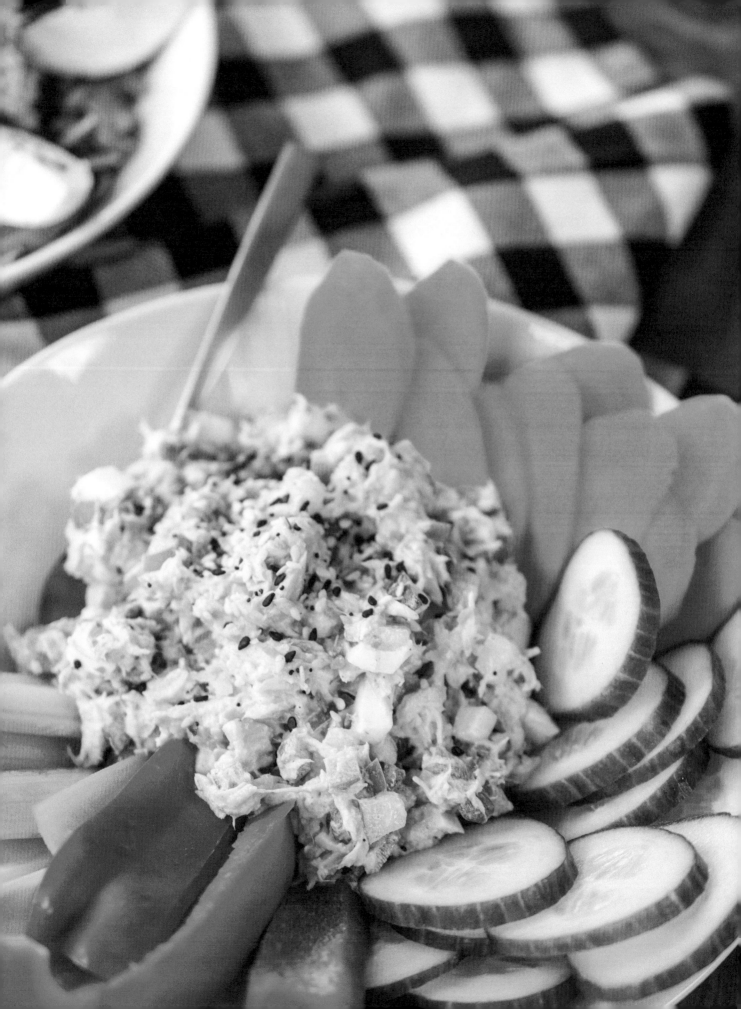

CHUNG'S POKE BOWL

Chung Chow, Food Stylist

Rivals the restaurants. Period.

Ingredients

2 tablespoons soy sauce

1 teaspoon rice wine vinegar

1 teaspoon sesame oil

1 tablespoon finely chopped green onion

¼ teaspoon roasted sesame seeds

1 cup sushi-grade tuna, cubed

Brown Rice

Toppings: sesame seeds, cucumber, everything bagel seasoning, shredded nori (a type of dried seaweed), wasabi—on the side

Directions

1. In a large bowl, mix together soy sauce, rice wine vinegar, sesame oil, green onions, and roasted sesame seeds.

2. Add cubed tuna, toss to coat. Cover and refrigerate for 15 minutes to 1 hour.

3. Cook rice according to package directions.

4. Add brown rice to the bottom of a serving bowl, top with tuna, and the toppings of your choice.

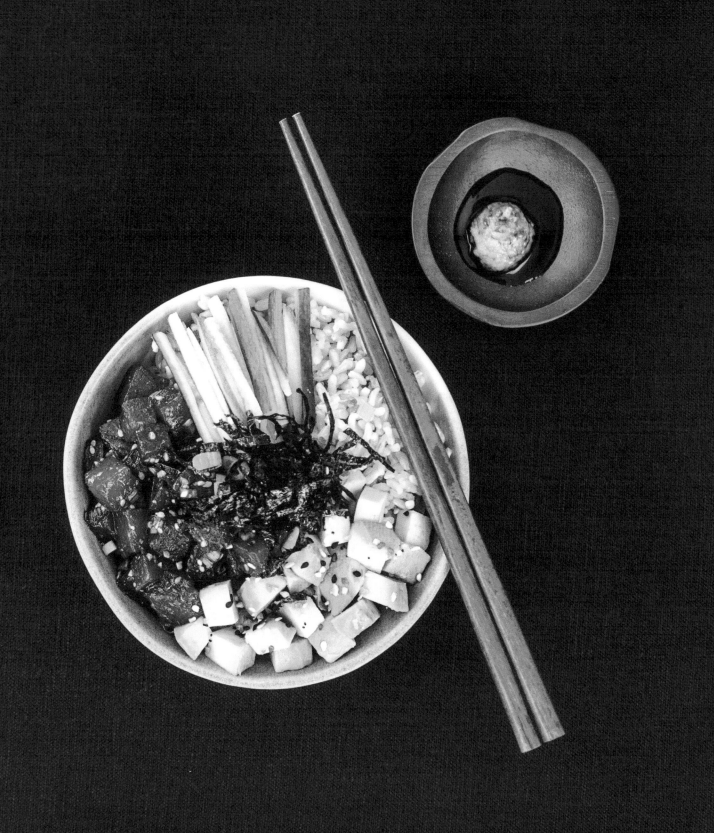

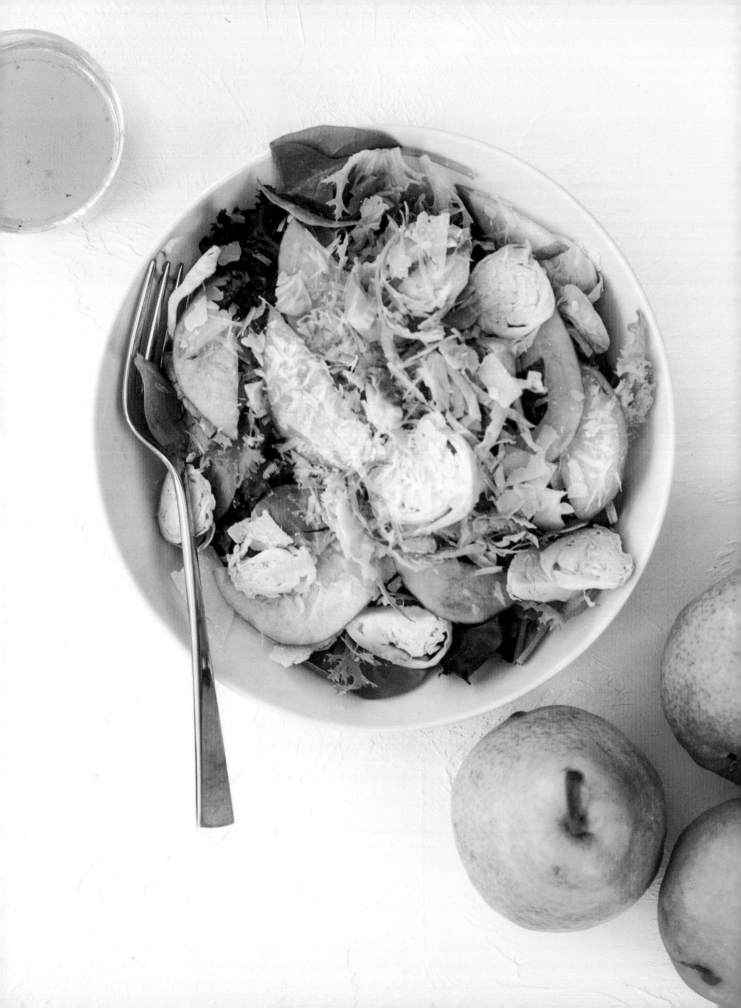

MEGAN'S BRUSSELS, PEAR, AND PARM SALAD

Megan Wilcop, Graphic Designer

Light. Fresh. And beyond delish.

Ingredients

¼ cup olive oil

1 tablespoon white wine vinegar

2 tablespoons honey

Juice of one lemon

Pears

Brussels sprouts, shredded

Spring Mix

Parmesan cheese, shaved

Directions

1. In a small bowl, make the dressing by whisking together olive oil, white wine vinegar, honey, and lemon juice.

2. Slice pears into bite-size pieces.

3. Top spring mix with brussels sprouts and pears. Drizzle with dressing and top with parm.

Beth's Tip

Need a protein boost? Add roasted chicken sausage to this beauty.

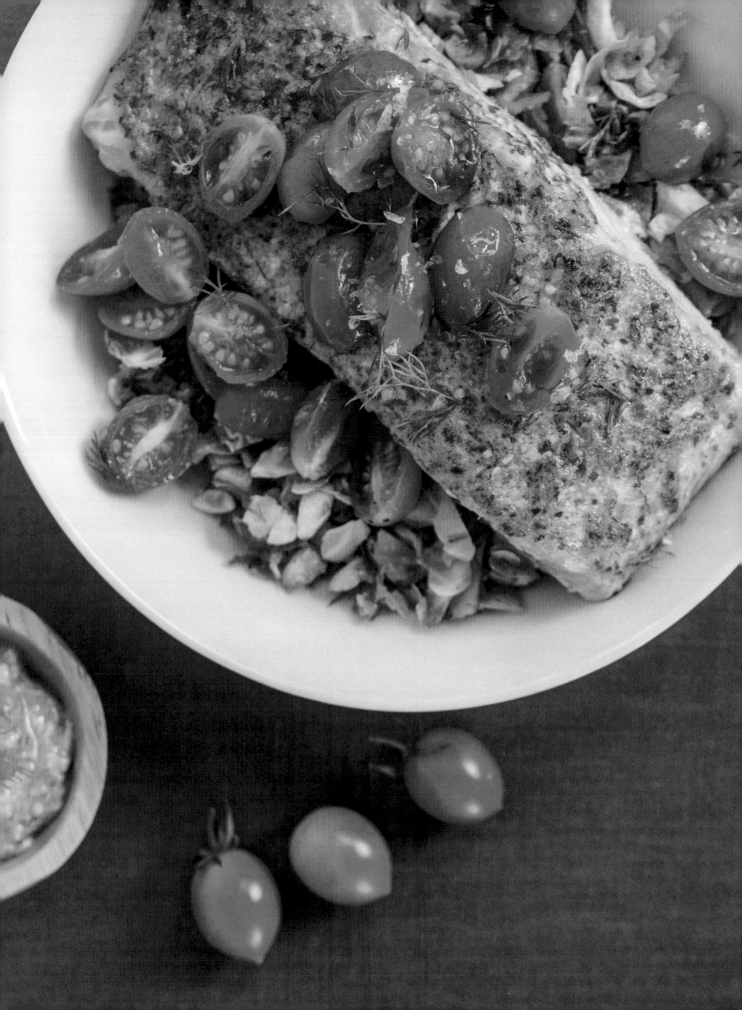

ANGELA'S ONE PAN PESTO SALMON
WITH TOMATOES AND BRUSSELS

Angela McColgin, Editor

All. The. Yes. And she's #lowcarb.

Ingredients

4 (6 to 8-ounce) salmon fillets

8 tablespoons butter

4 tablespoons pesto

1 tablespoon freshly chopped dill

Cherry or grape tomatoes

Olive oil

Salt and pepper

Brussels sprouts, shredded

Everything bagel seasoning

Directions

1. Preheat oven to 400° F and line a baking sheet with foil.

2. In a small bowl, make pesto butter by combining softened butter, pesto, and dill. Stir together until smooth.

3. Place salmon fillets on one end of the baking sheet. Season with salt and pepper. Top each fillet with a scoop of pesto butter and smooth over the top.

4. Cut tomatoes in half. Toss with olive oil. Season with salt and pepper. Place tomatoes next to the salmon down the center of the baking sheet.

5. Toss shredded brussels sprouts with olive oil. Season with salt, pepper, and bagel seasoning. Place sprouts next to tomatoes on the end of the baking sheet opposite the salmon.

6. Roast everything for 25-30 minutes, until the salmon is cooked through and flakes easily with a fork.

7. Serve salmon on top of brussels sprouts. Top with roasted tomatoes.

RUTHIE'S STUFFED PEPPERS

Shelly Ruth, Photography

Fiery, with lots of flavorful attitude, just like Ruthie.

Ingredients

4 bell peppers

Quinoa

½ pound ground turkey

½ pound ground sirloin

Taco seasoning

Toppings: black beans, salsa verde, feta cheese, greek yogurt, chili lime, tortilla chips

Directions

1. Preheat oven to 425°F and line a baking sheet with foil.

2. Prepare peppers by slicing off the tops and scooping out the guts. Set aside.

3. Prepare quinoa according to package directions.

4. In a skillet over medium heat, brown turkey and beef. Season with taco seasoning.

5. Add cooked quinoa to the ground meat mixture. Stir to combine.

6. Spoon an equal amount of the meat mixture into each pepper and place them on the baking sheet.

7. Bake peppers for 25 minutes.

8. While peppers are baking, heat black beans.

9. Remove peppers from the oven, top with black beans, salsa, feta, greek yogurt, and a dash of chili lime. Serve tortilla chips on the side.

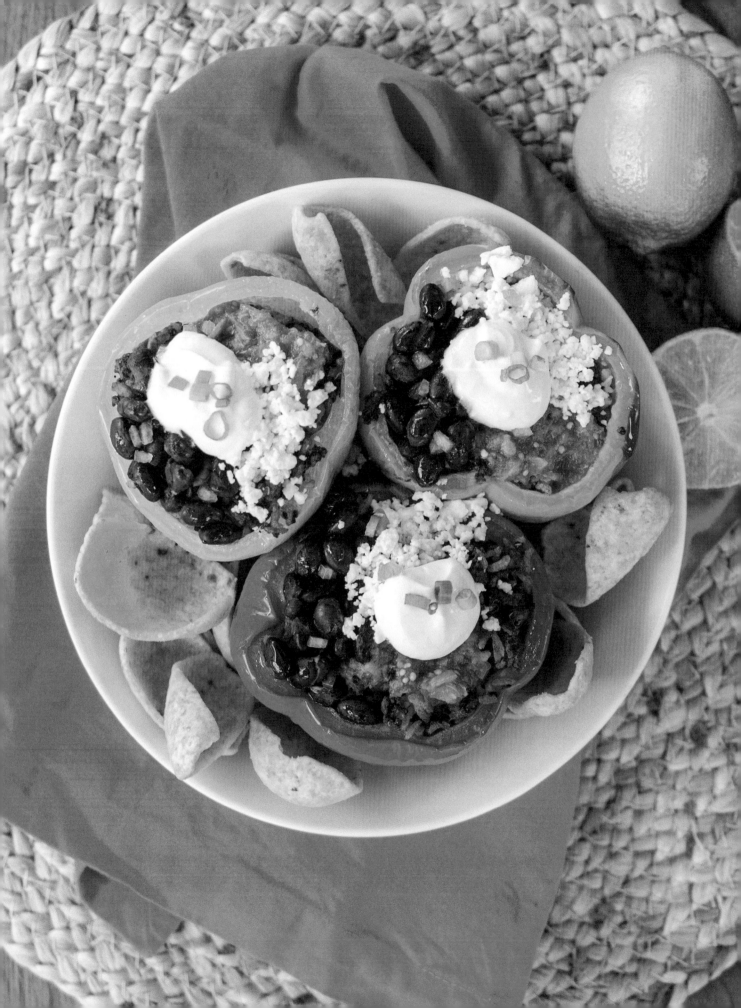

LOW-CARB EATS

BOWLS + MEALS

All Day Everyday Arugula, 19
Angela's One Pan Pesto Salmon with
Roasted Tomatoes and Brussels, 157
Ashley's Salmon Salad, 150
Aunt Kitty Salad, 37
Black and Blue Bowl, 20
Buffalo Blue Turkey Burger, 25
Egg Muffins, 86
Eggplant Parm Stacks, 22
Grilled Cauliflower with Avocado
Salsa Verde, 93
Johnny's Filets, 81
Parmesan Crusted Salmon, 31
Pesto Chicken Cauliflower Pizza, 32
Roasted Veggie Bowl, 41
Salsa Verde Chicken, 34
Seersucker Chicken, 16
Shaved Brussels with Bacon and Egg, 42
Shrimp and Cauliflower Grits, 28
Spaghetti Squash with Pesto
  and Tomatoes, 38
That Egg Roll Bowl, 26

SNACKS

Bacon and Peanut Butter, 96

DRINKS

Chocolate Peanut Butter Protein Shake, 124
Low-Carb Moscow Mule, 110
Spicy Paloma, 109

REGULAR MACRO EATS

RECIPE INDEX

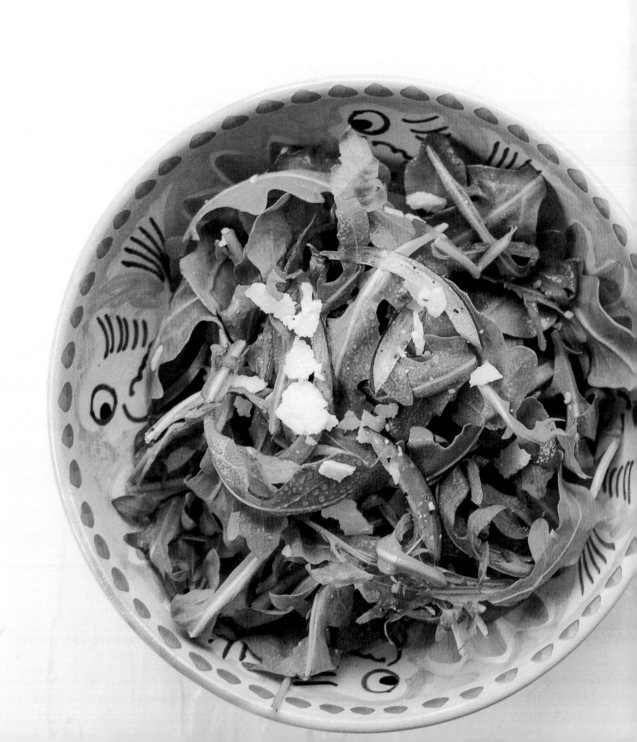

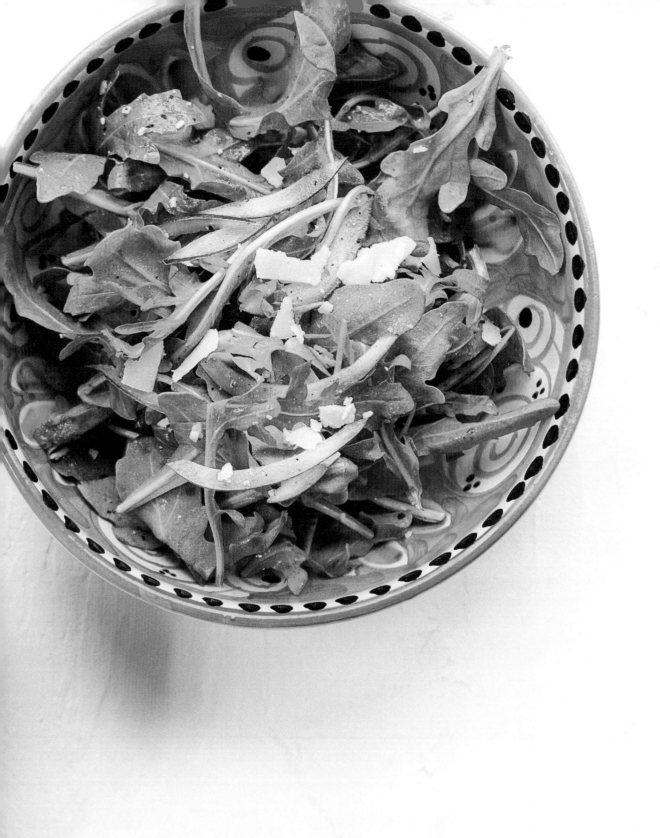

ACKNOWLEDGMENTS

First and foremost, to my family: John, Chase, Campbell, and Calvin. You all are a constant source of strength, support, inspiration, love, and just the best bunch of cheerleaders a gal could ever hope for. Thank you for loving me unconditionally always. I hope I made you proud, and I hope we can pass this book down to your kiddos someday. Also, thank you for eating more rice and chicken bowls than is probably acceptable. #seedsofchange I love you forever and ever.

To the Brunch'd team—Ashley, Shelly, Angela, and Megan—wowza! We did it, you crazy hooligans! Thank you for your time, commitment, devotion, support, motivation—laughs—oh, the list goes on. Your talents are forever appreciated, girls. Thank you for taking a chance on me and helping me bring this baby to life. I adore you all.

To our sweet and beautiful Chung, thank you, thank you for helping bring my vision to life and then adding your gorgeous twists. What a talented gem you are. Can't wait to cook up something else with you.

To my parents, thank you for always believing in me and teaching me "the sky is the limit" and to "never be afraid to march to the beat of my own drum." Your children and grandchildren are beyond blessed that you are all ours! Oh, and thank you for continuing to laugh at the thought of me being a cook. Your motivation tactics are interesting at best, but they work.

To the Seersucker readers, man, where do I begin? It's safe to say this little cooking stint would not be in existence without you all. Eight years of support from you led me to this point, and I'm truly forever grateful for our community. Thank you for the journey, gang. It's been the most remarkable ride. You've made it a great one.

Xx.

beth.

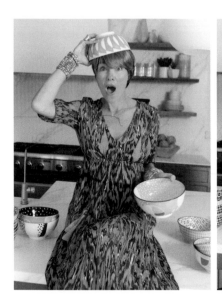
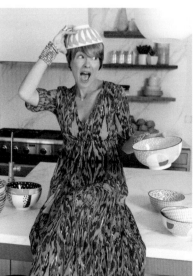
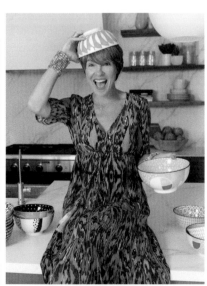

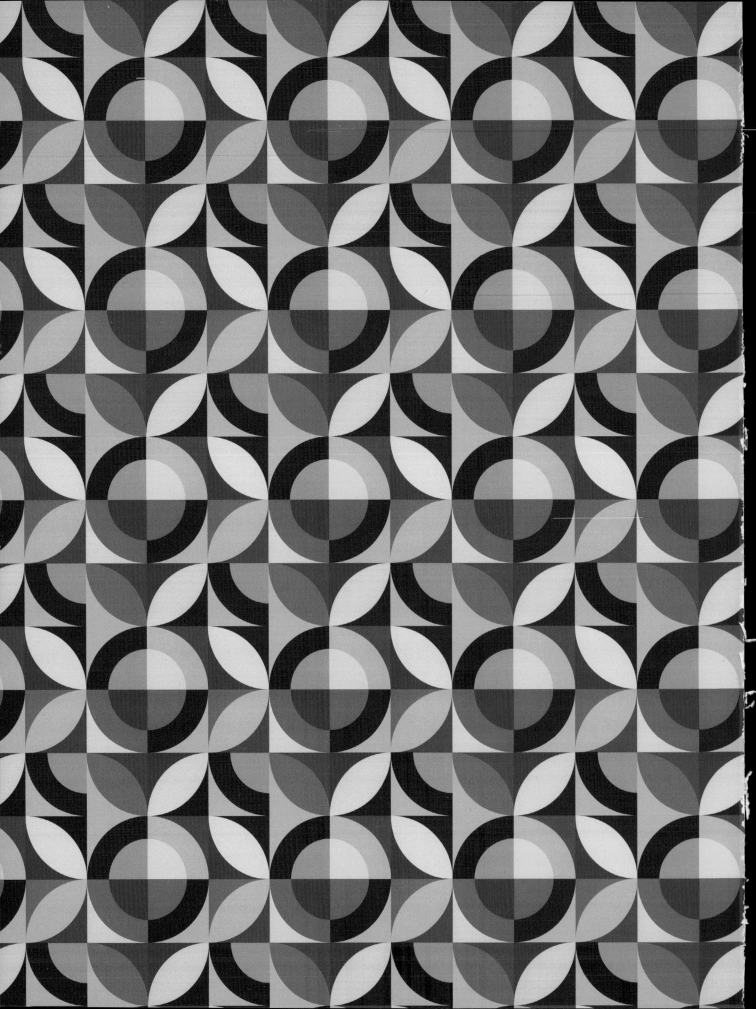